Schriftenreihe Neurologie –

17

Takayuki Tsuboi · Walter Christian

EPILEPSY

*A Clinical, Electroencephalographic, and Statistical
Study of 466 Patients*

With 11 Figures

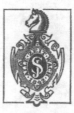

Springer-Verlag Berlin · Heidelberg · New York 1976

Privatdozent Dr. TAKAYUKI TSUBOI
Institute of Anthropology and Human Genetics
University of Heidelberg

now:
Professor Dr. TAKAYUKI TSUBOI
Tokyo Metropolitan Institute for Neurosciences
2—6 Musashidai, Fuchu-City,
Tokyo, Japan

Professor Dr. WALTER CHRISTIAN
Department of Neurology
University of Heidelberg

ISBN-13: 978-3-642-66376-5   e-ISBN-13: 978-3-642-66374-1
DOI: 10.1007/978-3-642-66374-1

Library of Congress Cataloging in Publication Data. Tsuboi, Takayuki, 1931— Epilepsy : a clinical, electro-encephalographic, and statistical study of 466 patients. (Neurology series ; no 17) Includes bibliographical references and index. 1. Epilepsy—Cases, clinical reports, statistics. I. Christian, Walter, joint author. II. Title. III. Series: Schriftenreihe neurologie ; no. 17. [DNLM: 1. Epilepsy. Wl SC344 Bd. 17 / WL385 T882e 1976] RC372.T77 616.8'53'09 76-13053

Offsetprinting and bookbinding: Konrad Triltsch, Graphischer Betrieb, 87 Würzburg.

Contents

Introduction

Although a number of studies have addressed epilepsy from a variety of qualitative and quantitative factors, relatively little systematic or multidisciplinary work has been reported to date. The general purpose of the present study was to analyze specific kinds of data from a large series of epileptic patients to focus the significance of the findings, particularly in relation to previously published results. Correlations among the following parameters are presented: age, sex, age at onset of seizure, type of seizure, paroxysmal electroencephalogram (EEG) abnormalities, basic EEG rhythm, family predisposition to epilepsy, and the presence of exogenous factors.

The basic material of the present study consists of records of approximately 7400 patients treated at the outpatient clinic of the Department of Neurology, University of Heidelberg, in whom the clinical diagnosis suggested some type of epilepsy. Initially, the first consecutive 500 patients in an alphabetically arranged file were chosen for inclusion within the study if their clinical diagnosis was supplemented by at least one EEG examination. The final study group consisted of 466 patients, since 34 patients had to be excluded because of the lack of sufficient clinical information concerning them.

The statistical analysis presented includes the χ^2 test, Fisher's exact test, Student's t test, and coefficient of contingency analysis. In cases where the differences are statistically significant, the terms <u>increase</u> or <u>decrease</u> are used. For instances where evidence for a significant difference was obtained, the expression <u>higher</u> or <u>lower</u> frequency is applied.

Results and Discussion

I. Age

1. Distribution by Age

The ages of the total number of patients ranged from 5 - 78 years, as shown in Table 1. The highest rate of incidence of epilepsy was seen in the age group 20 - 24 years (17 %). Most patients were within the age range 10 - 44 years (390 patients, 84 %). The age distribution of female patients was slightly younger than that of male patients.

2. Age and Sex

Sex distribution varied in the various age groups, as shown in Table 1. Among the young patients, males were predominant; but a reverse tendency was noted in the aged epileptics. This will be discussed later because it may be correlated with the age at onset of disease and with type of seizure in some instances.

3. Young, Adult, and Aged Patients, and Their Correlated Findings

The patients were divided into three groups according to age: young patients, 19 years or younger (121 patients or 26 %), adult patients, those between 20 and 49 years (304 patients or 65 %), and aged patients, 50 years or over (41 patients or 8.8 %). Distribution by sex, type of seizure (grand mal (GM) or petit mal (PM)), α-EEG, β-EEG, and focal sign in EEG in the three age groups is shown in Table 2.

Compared with the older age patients (adult and aged patients), young patients showed a higher frequency of awakening grand mal and less grand mal during sleep as well as diffuse grand mal. In addition an increased frequency of patients with absence petit mal (22 % : 12.5 % or 43 of 345, $P < 0.01$) and those with total petit mal (35 %, $P < 0.001$) was found. The young patients also showed an increased frequency of patients with paroxysmal EEG abnormalities (74 %, $P < 0.001$), spike-and-wave complex (sp-w-c) (27 %, $P < 0.001$), abnormal EEG (55 %, $P < 0.01$), slow waves (slow wave dominant EEG) (50 %, $P < 0.001$), pathologic changes during hyperventilation (42 %, $P < 0.01$), and an increased family predisposition to the disease (18 %, $P < 0.001$), as indicated by a sign (increase ↑ or decrease ↓) in Table 2.

Compared with the younger age patients (young and adult patients), aged patients showed an increased frequency of patients with grand mal during sleep (37 %, P < 0.01) and those with psycho-motor epilepsy (44 %, P < 0.01). A decreased frequency of patients with awakening grand mal (17 %, P < 0.05), myoclonic petit mal (0 %, P(Fisher) = 0.035), total petit mal (7 %, P < 0.05), and with cortical epilepsy (0 %, P(Fisher) = 0.021) and the presence of exogenous factors (2.4 %, P(Fisher) = 0.021) was also observed in this group.

As shown in Table 2, the findings in adult patients were intermediate to those in the young and those in the aged groups. A characteristic finding was the increase of male patients (63 %, P < 0.05). The low voltage EEG was found only in this age group (P(Fisher) = 0.004).

Comparison of the two age groups of young and adult, and adult patients revealed a statistically significant difference, as indicated by an unequal sign (> or <) in Table 2.

4. Correlation Between Age and Other Factors

Significant correlations were found between age and (1) the occurrence of paroxysmal and other EEG abnormalities, (2) basic EEG rhythm, (3) family predisposition to the disease (incidence of patients with epileptic relatives of the first or second degrees) and (4) exogenous factors, which include perinatal and postnatal brain damages such as birth injuries, encephalitis, head trauma, etc., as shown in Table 2.

Correlation between age, sex, and other factors is analyzed and discussed in detail in Chapter II.

5. Discussion and Summary

A total of 466 patients were divided into three age groups, and age-correlated factors were analyzed. The three age groups demonstrated their different characteristic findings, that is, young patients under 19 years showed a high frequency of patients with awakening grand mal, absence petit mal, paroxysmal EEG abnormalities, especially sp-w-c, slow wave dominant EEG in basic rhythm, pathologic changes during hyperventilation, and family predisposition, and less grand mal during sleep, as well as diffuse grand mal. Aged patients over 50 years of age revealed different findings from those in the young patients, while the results for adult patients were intermediate to those for the young and aged patients.

A correlation between age and type of seizure was roughly analyzed by BOLDYREV (1970), RODRIGO LONDONO (1969), BONDEULLE et al. (1970), HORI (1960), HOPKINS (1933), and others. Younger patients aged 10 - 14 years showed the highest frequency of sp-w-c abnormality and in the total EEG abnormalities, irrespective of idiopathic or symptomatic pathogenesis (ROBINSON and OSTERHELD, 1947). These results were confirmed in repeated EEG examinations by AJMONE MARSAN and ZIVIN (1970) in 308 epileptic patients, and also in psychopathic, schizophrenic patients and in normal control subjects (HILL, 1952). In younger patients, LUNDERVOLD et al. (1959) observed more 3/s sp-w-c, focal, as well as background abnormalities, while older patients showed more normal background activities. LENNOX and DAVIS (1950) analyzed a correlation between age and 3/s- or 2/s sp-w-c and found that younger patients aged 1 - 4 years frequently showed 2/s sp-w-c, and patients aged 5 - 12 years showed a similar frequency distribution, while patients over 13 years revealed more frequent 3/s sp-w-c. A correlation between age and basic EEG rhythm was systematically examined by PETERSEN and EEG OLOFSSON (1971), and they reported that epileptic patients under 10 years showed an increased incidence of theta dominant basic rhythm. Other age-correlated factors were found, such as α-rhythm (PETERSEN and EEG OLOFSSON, 1971; the increase of α-frequency linearly with age), β-EEG (GIBBS et al., 1943; the higher incidence of β-EEG in adults than in children, especially in the aged female patients, VOGEL and GÖTZE, 1962), θ waves (HILL, 1952; EEG OLOFSSON, 1970; MUNDY-CASTLE, 1951; the highest incidence of slow waves in patients 5 - 7 years of age, decreasing after that age, a lower incidence among aged subjects), focal abnormalities (LUNDERVOLD et al., 1959; HUGHES, 1967; aged subjects and children were apt to have focal abnormalities, GIBBS and GIBBS, 1952; NIEDERMEYER, 1957). Family predisposition and exogenous factors, as an etiology for epilepsy, were found to be correlated with age and age at onset of seizure as well (BUENO et al., 1970). Among aged patients, the relative importance of exogenous factors has been suggested (GÄNSHIRT, 1970).

Thus, the striking age-correlated results observed in the present study are supported by those of previous studies. All the previous authors analyzed these correlations from limited viewpoints, while the present authors have analyzed these from as many viewpoints as possible. Some authors, however, have found different age correlations from those of the present study. MATTHES (1970) found no age correlation in grand mal, cortical, or psychomotor epilepsy among children; GLASER and GOLUB (1955) found no correlation between age and paroxysmal EEG abnormalities.

II. Sex

A sex ratio in a total patient sample depends on sampling methods, age, type of seizure, EEG, family predisposition, and the presence of exogenous factors of the patients studied. Correlation between sex and these factors should be analyzed.

1. Sex and Age at Onset of Seizure

The frequency of patients with onset of seizure at 2 - 9 years was higher in female patients (30 % vs. 19 %, P < 0.01) than in

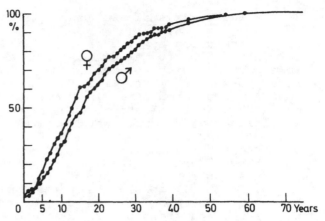

Fig. 1. Accumulative frequency of age at onset of seizure

males. Age at onset was somewhat earlier in female than in male
patients, as shown in Table 3 and Figure 1. The mean age at onset
in male patients was 18.7 years and in female patients 17.0 years.
The difference is not statistically significant. However, when
all patients were ranked according to age at onset of disease
as in Tables 11 and 12, onset of disease was earlier in male
than in female patients only when it occurred in early childhood.

This fact may be connected with the finding that the main types
of seizure occurring in early childhood were the West and Lennox
syndromes which affect predominantly males. The presence of exogenous factors or a positive family history for epilepsy is also
more common in patients with these syndromes. Perinatal and postnatal brain damage was more frequently seen in male babies, which
might also be a related factor. As shown in the next chapter,
males are more prone to late-onset epilepsy than females (KUHLO
and SCHWARZ, 1971).

2. Sex and Type of Seizure

Correlations between sex and type of seizure are shown in Table 4.
The distribution by type of seizure was similar in both sexes
except that the frequency of total petit mal was higher in female
than male patients (27 % vs. 20 %, P < 0.05). A higher frequency
of patients with absence petit mal and those of psychomotor epilepsy and a lower frequency of patients with cortical epilepsy
were seen in females. In male patients, pure type of seizure
(54 % in males vs. 43 % in females) was increased (P < 0.05)
compared with the incidence in females. However, the frequency
of other pure types of seizure did not differ between the sexes
(Table 5).

In this study, absence and total petit mal as well as psychomotor
epilepsy were more common in female patients, whereas cortical
epilepsy was detected in a higher proportion of male patients.
These correlations will be discussed in detail in Chapter III.

3. Sex and Paroxysmal EEG Abnormalities

The distribution by type of paroxysmal EEG abnormality is shown in Table 6. The frequency was increased more in female than in male patients with atypical sp-w-c (16 % vs. 8 %, P < 0.01) and total sp-w-c (22 % vs. 12 %, P < 0.01). The frequency of total paroxysmal abnormalities in female patients was higher than in male (63 % in females : 57 % in males). However no statistically significant differences were found.

The frequency of individual types of paroxysmal activity is shown in Tables 17 and 18. The increased frequency in female over male patients was found only in these with 3.5-5/s sp-w-c (13 % vs. 3.6 %, P < 0.01) and in these with multiple sp-w-c (16 % vs. 8.7 %, P < 0.05). The abnormal EEG characteristic of epilepsy was found with increased frequency in female over male patients (23 % vs. 13 %, P < 0.01, Table 7).

In previous studies, a higher frequency of EEG abnormality has been reported among female than male patients (O'BRIEN et al., 1959). In the present study, the authors did not find a difference between the sexes in the occurrence of paroxysmal EEG abnormalities. However, sp-w-c and pathognomonic evidence of typical EEG patterns were more common in female than in male patients. Marked differences in atypical-, 3.5-5/s-, multiple-, and total sp-w-c (more common in females) were also found in the present study.

4. Sex and Basic EEG Rhythm (Table 7)

4.1. α-EEG

The present study revealed that female patients have an increased incidence of high voltage α-rhythm compared to male patients (15 % : 7 %, P < 0.01). However, DIEKER (1967) found no sex difference in the incidence of high voltage α-rhythm among family members of twin probands. The incidence of high voltage α-rhythm detected in the present study (10 %) was higher than that in the general population as published by DIEKER (1967, 4.3 %). According to PETERSEN and EEG OLOFSSON (1971), girls showed a higher frequency of α-rhythm than boys. This correlation was not analyzed in our study.

4.2. β-EEG

The incidence of β-EEG was increased more in female than in male patients (23 % for females : 14 % for males, P < 0.05). The incidence of β-EEG was increased in healthy females (62 % for females, 43 % for males) a finding also reported by MUNDY-CASTLE (1951). VOGEL and GÖTZE (1962) also found a higher incidence of β-EEG among adult female patients (13 % vs. 8.5 %), especially female patients over 35 years, and an even greater incidence among those over 45 years of age.

4.3. Slow Waves, Low Voltage EEG, Pathologic Findings During Hyperventilation and Focal Sign

In the present study, no marked differences were found between males and females in the incidence of slow waves (slow wave dominant basic rhythm), low voltage EEG (below 20 µV in all leads), pathologic findings during hyperventilation or focal sign. Although PETERSEN and EEG OLOFSSON (1971) found slow waves at the occipital area more common among girls, they reported no data with respect to low voltage EEG or pathologic findings during hyperventilation. In studies of epileptic children, RICCI and SCARINCI (1963) found a predominance of focal epileptic EEG abnormality in boys (56 %).

5. Sex and Familial Predisposition (Table 8)

The frequency of patients with familial predisposition to epilepsy was slightly higher in male patients compared to females. Conversely, among girls with pure petit mal, CURRIER et al. (1963) found a higher frequency of familial predisposition, especially on the maternal side. In the present study, the authors observed that a correlation existed between the frequency of familial predisposition and age, age of onset, type of seizure, and EEG and the presence of exogenous factors. The authors also observed an increased frequency of familial predisposition among female patients with petit mal as will be discussed in the next chapter.

6. Sex and Exogenous Factors (Table 8)

Male patients showed a higher frequency of exogenous factors than did females (17 % for males, 6.3 % for females, $P < 0.001$). In particular, a significant increase was found in male patients with very early onset (0 - 1 year, 29 %) and in those with onset between 20 and 39 years (29 %, see Table 36).

7. Discussion and Summary

The sex ratios for various types of seizure for our cases differed from those reported in previous studies. In general, however, just as in previous studies, some types of seizures were found predominantly in males, while other types were found more often in females. Very different characteristic patterns in distribution of patients by age at onset of seizure in the two sexes have been shown in this Chapter (III.3) and illustrated in Figure 2a-f. Male predominance at the age of onset at 0 - 1 year may be correlated with a higher frequency of West syndrome and of Lennox syndrome, and later development of psychomotor epilepsy, and with exogenous factors in this age range. Female predominance at prepuberty as well as at puberty may be correlated with a higher frequency of absence petit mal in this age range. Among those in whom seizures began at a later age, more male patients

were found in the present study than in previous studies (KUHLO
and SCHWARZ, 1971; MAYER and TRÜBESTEIN, 1968; NIEDERMEYER, 1958).
In our study, female patients revealed a higher frequency of EEG
abnormalities than reported by O'BRIEN et al. (1959) among others,
especially in atypical, 3.5-5/s, and multiple sp-w-c. In basic EEG
rhythm, female patients demonstrated β-EEG in a higher incidence
than found by MUNDY-CASTLE (1951). An increased frequency of
familial predisposition in female patients with petit mal as
found by CURRIER et al. (1963) and that of exogenous factors in
boys were also observed in the present study.

Thus, nearly all the previously reported characteristic findings
in male as well as in female patients were confirmed in the present study by multidisciplinary analyses.

Correlations between sex and other factors have been analyzed in
this chapter. Females comprised 40.8 % of our patients. Compared
to male patients, they were younger, showed an earlier onset of
seizure, and an increased frequency of total petit mal, absence
PM, combined type of seizure, atypical sp-w-c, 3.5-5/s sp-w-c,
multiple sp-w-c, and EEG abnormalities characteristic of epilepsy,
and a decreased frequency of cortical epilepsy. In the basic EEG
rhythm, female patients showed an increased frequency of high
voltage α- and β-EEG compared to male patients. The frequency
of familial predisposition and the presence of exogenous factors
were higher in male than in female patients.

III. Type of Seizure

The description and classification of the various clinical types
of seizure are based on that defined by JANZ (1969); however,
only the following ten clinical types of seizure have been selected for use by the authors in this study.

Grand mal

    1. Awakening grand mal (A-GM)
    2. Grand mal during sleep (S-GM)·
    3. Diffuse grand mal (D-GM)
    4. Occasional grand mal (O-GM)

Petit mal

    5. West syndrome (Blitz-Nick-Salaam-Krämpfe, infantile
       spasm, propulsive petit mal)
    6. Lennox syndrome (myoclonic astatic petit mal)
    7. Absence petit mal (petit mal, pure petit mal)
    8. Myoclonic petit mal (myoclonic epilepsy, impulsive
       petit mal)
    9. Psychomotor epilepsy
  10. Cortical epilepsy (focal epilepsy)

Other types (including febrile convulsions, epileptic equivalent,
syncopal attack, etc.) have been excluded from consideration be-

cause they represent only a small part of the total types of
seizure occurring in the patients (33 of a total of 699 seizures, 4.7 %).

Distribution of patients by type of seizure is indicated in Table
4. The majority of patients exhibited grand mal; 23 % of all patients had petit mal and 26 % psychomotor epilepsy. Of those
with grand mal, awakening grand mal was most common (32 %); absence petit mal was the most common finding in patients with
petit mal. Two hundred and thirty patients (49 %) had a pure
type of seizure (only one clinical type of seizure); the re-
maining 236 patients (51 %) had combined types of seizures. Petit
mal was more prone to be of a combined type than grand mal (the
proportion of combined types of PM was 87 % or 90 of 106, and
that of GM 54 % or 203 of 375; see Table 5, P < 0.001). Psychomotor epilepsy had a similar tendency (the combined proportion
is 80 % or 95 of 119, P < 0.001). Grand mal and cortical epilepsy
were less commonly associated with combined-type seizures (54 %
and 55 %, respectively). Female patients were found to have an
increased frequency of a combined type of grand mal than males
(62 % for females and 49 % for males, P < 0.05), compared to the
total number of patients (43 % for females, 54 % for males, P <
0.05, Table 5).

The high frequency of combined types of seizures in the present
study corresponds to the figure of 65 % in Medical World News
(1970) which stated that the frequency of more than one type of
seizure seems to be much higher than previously assumed.

With respect to the incidence of each type of seizure, various
authors cite very different figures. Concerning the frequency
distribution of awakening, sleep, and diffuse grand mal, the
present study shows a greater frequency of awakening grand mal
than reported in previous studies. However, the frequency of
grand mal during sleep was lower than that reported by JANZ (1969)
and by FURUICHI (1969), but higher than that observed by KRISCHEK
(1962). In comparison with previous studies, a higher frequency
of absence PM, myoclonic PM, and total GM was observed. The validity of such conclusions depends, however, on many factors,
including sampling methods (selected or unselected patients),
age range, sex, diagnostic criteria, observation period, race,
etc. As shown in Table 2, the distribution of patients by age
was found in this study to correlate with type of seizure. This
correlation is analyzed in detail in the next section.

1. Type of Seizure and Age

The correlation between type of seizure and current age is shown
in Tables 9 and 10.

1.1. Male Patients

A higher frequency of patients with A-GM (42 % or 37 of 88 patients, P < 0.01) was observed in the age group 15 - 24 years,

a higher frequency of S-GM (28 % or 24 of 87 patients, P < O.05)
in patients over 35 years; a higher frequency of absence PM in
patients 5 - 24 years (21 % or 25 of 120 patients, P < O.001), a
higher frequency of total PM in patients 5 - 24 years (31 % or
37 of 120 patients, P < O.001), and a higher frequency of psychomotor epilepsy in patients over 50 years (45 % or 9 of 20 patients, P < O.001).

1.2. Female Patients

A higher frequency of A-GM (52 % or 16 of 31 patients, P < O.05)
was observed in patients aged 15 - 19 years; a higher frequency
of S-GM (39 % or 12 of 31 patients, P < O.01) in patients over
45 years; a higher frequency of D-GM (29 % or 12 of 41 patients,
P < O.05) in patients 30 - 39 years; a higher frequency of myoclonic PM (16 % or 17 of 108 patients, P < O.01) in patients 15 - 34
years; and a higher frequency of total PM (35 % or 28 of 80 patients, P < O.05) in patients 5 - 24 years.

1.3. Total Patients

The frequency of A-GM (42 % or 60 of 144 patients, P < O.01) observed showed an increase in the age group 15 - 24 years; an increased frequency of S-GM (34 % or 21 of 62 patients, P < O.01)
in patients over 45 years; an increased frequency of D-GM (21 %,
P < O.01) in patients over 35 years; an increased frequency of
absence PM (22 %, P < O.001) in patients 5 - 24 years; an increased frequency of myoclonic PM (9.8 %, P < O.01) in patients
10 - 39 years; and an increased frequency of total PM (29 %, P <
O.001) in patients 5 - 29 years. These results indicate a close
correlation between type of seizure and age. Certain types of
seizure were very commonly seen in a given age range and could
be correlated with age at onset of seizure.

Correlations between type of seizure and age have been previously
analyzed by various authors. Some types of seizure frequently
occurred within a certain age range, as described by JANZ (1969)
among others. Petit mal and grand mal were found more frequently
among children, whereas psychomotor epilepsy as well as cortical
seizure were observed more frequently in adults (GOMES LINS and
FARIAS DA SILVA, 1969).

When the frequencies of seizure type between children and adults
were compared, the difference was clearly evident.

A difference in frequency of type of grand mal was also observed
to vary according to age. There was a higher frequency of awakening grand mal and a lower frequency of diurnal grand mal among
children under 16 years of age than among adults. However, no
difference was found in those with nocturnal grand mal (HOPKINS,
1933). HORI (1959) reported an increased frequency of myoclonic
petit mal among younger patients (under 14 years of age) with
multiple sp-w-c EEG.

A difference in frequency of seizure was found not only between children and adults but also between infant and aged epileptics. RODRIGO LONDONO (1969) frequently found grand mal, hemi-grand mal, and West syndrome in patients aged 0 - 1 year old and an absence of myoclonic petit mal and automatism in patients between 2 and 12 years of age at onset. However, MATTHES (1970) found no age correlation among children with grand mal, or with cortical or psychomotor epilepsy. Among aged patients, BONDUELLA et al. (1970), among others, frequently found grand mal and cortical epilepsy.

There was a difference of frequency in type of seizure occurring among young, adult, and aged patients as indicated in Table 2. In young patients, the frequency of awakening grand mal was higher, whereas that of grand mal during sleep was found only infrequently, as reported by HOPKINS (1933). In our study, absence and total petit mal occurred more often in this age group. The frequency of myoclonic petit mal was higher than that found by HORI (1959). In the present study, aged patients were found to have an increased frequency of grand mal during sleep and of psychomotor epilepsy, whereas the frequency of awakening grand mal, myoclonic petit mal, total petit mal, and of cortical epilepsy was lower.

As shown in Table 5, 230 patients (49 %) revealed a pure type of seizure. This frequency was lower than that reported in children by BAMBERGER and MATTHES (1959) (209/349, 60 %) (P < 0.01). This difference was attributed to a longer observation period of our adult patients. A comparison of frequencies of pure type in various types of seizures in child and adult epileptics revealed a significantly decreased frequency in West and Lennox syndromes in adults but an increased frequency of myoclonic PM as well as of psychomotor epilepsy. No difference in the frequency of grand mal and cortical epilepsy was found between children and adults.

2. Type of Seizure and Sex

The correlations between type of seizure and sex are shown in Table 4.

The frequency of absence PM, total PM, and psychomotor epilepsy in female patients was higher than in male patients. However, the difference was significant only in patients with total petit mal (18 % : 13 %, P < 0.05). In male patients, the frequency of cortical epilepsy was higher than in female patients, but not statistically significant. In all, the correlations in the two sexes were similar.

Male patients were predominantly found with West syndrome (BOWER and JEAVONS, 1959; BAMBERGER and MATTHES, 1959; MATTHES and MALLMANN-MÜHLBERGER, 1963; GASTAUT et al., 1964; JANZ, 1969); with Lennox syndrome (KRUSE, 1968; DOOSE, 1969; JANZ, 1969; SCHNEIDER et al., 1970); with psychomotor epilepsy (GLASER and GOLUB, 1955; BAMBERGER and MATTHES, 1959; JANZ, 1969); with cortical epilepsy (JANZ, 1969); and with grand mal (FURUICHI, 1969).

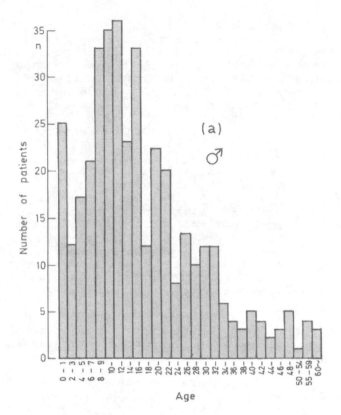

Fig. 2a. Age at onset of
seizure. Male patients

Female predominance was seen with pyknoleptic petit mal or absence petit mal (PACHE, 1952; LIVINGSTON, 1953; PAAL, 1957;
O'BRIEN et al., 1959; CURRIER et al., 1963; HERTOFT, 1963;
GIBBERD, 1963; MATTHES and WEBER, 1968; JANZ, 1969). Nearly the
same incidence in both sexes was found with myoclonic petit mal
(JANZ and CHRISTIAN, 1957); however, DALBY (1969) reported female predominance. Many authors did not identify sex ratio.

3. Type of Seizure and Age at Onset of Seizure

3.1. Male Patients

The distribution of male patients by age at onset of seizure is
shown in Table 11 and Figure 2a and 2b. The mean age at onset
was 18.7 ± S.E. 0.05 years. A higher frequency of A-GM was observed in the age group 6 - 17 years as well as that 6 - 22 years
($P < 0.01$ and $P < 0.001$, respectively); of D-GM in patients aged
0 - 4 years ($P < 0.01$); of absence PM in patients aged 4 - 17 years
($P < 0.001$); of myoclonic PM in patients aged 10 - 16 years ($P <
0.01$); of total PM in patients aged 4 - 17 years ($P < 0.001$); of
psychomotor epilepsy in patients aged 0 - 1 and 20 - 29 years ($P <
0.001$ and $P < 0.05$, respectively); and of cortical epilepsy in
patients aged 15 - 19 years ($P < 0.05$).

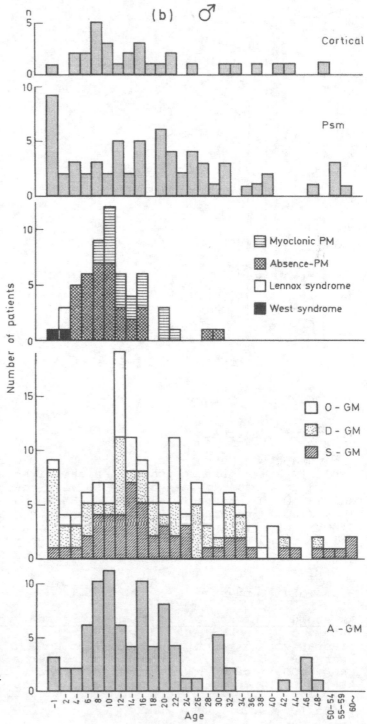

n
5
(b) ♂

Fig. 2b. Age at onset
and type of seizure.
Male patients

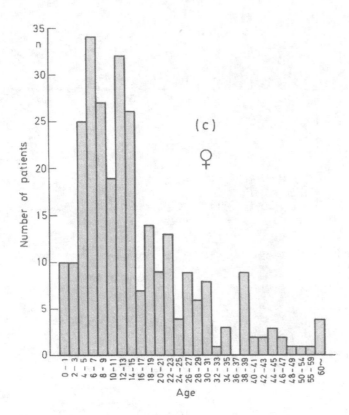

Fig. 2c. Age at onset of seizure. Female patients

3.2. Female Patients

The mean age at onset was 17.0 ± S.E. 0.07 years. As shown in Table 12 and Figure 2c and d, a higher frequency of A-GM was observed in the 5 - 15-year and 5 - 20-year age groups (P < 0.001 and P < 0.001, respectively), of S-GM in patients over 35 years (P < 0.001), of absence PM in patients aged 5 - 14 years (P < 0.001), of myoclonic PM in patients aged 12 - 15 years (P < 0.001), and of total PM in patients aged 4 - 15 years (P < 0.001).

3.3. Total Patients

As shown in Figure 2e and f, an increased frequency of A-GM was observed in 6 - 22-year-old patients (P < 0.001), of S-GM in patients over 35 years (P < 0.001), of D-GM in patients aged 0 - 4 years (P < 0.05), of absence PM in patients aged 5 - 12 years (P < 0.001), of myoclonic PM in patients aged 10 - 16 years (P < 0.001), of total PM in patients aged 5 - 17 years (P < 0.001), and of psychomotor epilepsy in patients aged 0 - 5 and 20 - 29 years (P < 0.001 and P < 0.05, respectively). The mean age at onset was 18.3 ± S.E. 0.03 years.

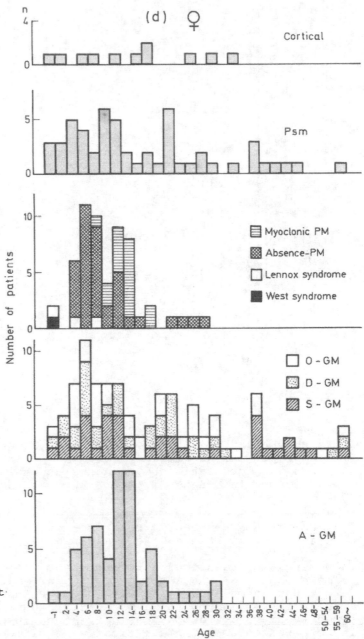

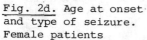

Fig. 2d. Age at onset and type of seizure. Female patients

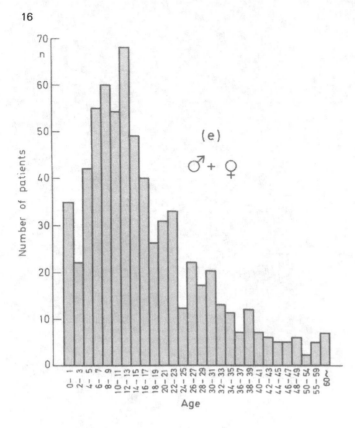

Fig. 2e. Age at onset of
seizure. Total patients

Certain types of seizures occurred more frequently within a given
age range as well as within a certain age range of onset as shown
in Table 13. Correlation between age at onset and type of seizure
are discussed in Chapter IV.9.

3.4. Comparison Between Correlations of Type of Seizure and Age at Onset in Male and Female Patients

In general, correlations between type of seizure and age at onset
in male and female patients were similar. Closer correlations
were found in male patients with D-GM, with psychomotor and cortical epilepsy, and with S-GM in female patients. Due to the
large standard deviation, the difference in the mean age at onset
in both sexes was not statistically significant. The significance
of age at onset of seizure will be discussed later in Chapter IV.

4. Type of Seizure and Paroxysmal EEG Abnormalities

Paroxysmal EEG abnormalities comprised of typical sp-w-c, atypical sp-w-c, sharp and slow waves, spikes, sharp waves, and temporal discharge are discussed in this section.

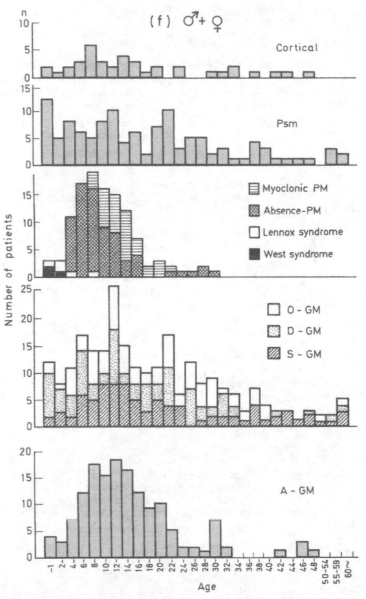

Fig. 2f. Age at onset and type of seizure. Total patients

Correlations between type of seizure and paroxysmal EEG abnormalities are shown in Tables 14 and 15 and Figure 3. In this section patients with certain types of seizure are compared with those with other types of seizure.

4.1. Male Patients (Table 14, Figure 3a)

4.1.1. Awakening Grand Mal

An increased frequency was observed in patients with 3/s sp-w-c (11 %, P < 0.05), in atypical sp-w-c (17 %, P < 0.001), in total sp-w-c (27 %, P < 0.001), and in total patients with paroxysmal abnormalities (71 %, P < 0.01).

4.1.2. Grand Mal During Sleep

A decreased frequency was found in patients with total sp-w-c (1.9 %, P < 0.05), and in total patients with paroxysmal abnormalities (42 %, P < 0.05).

4.1.3. Diffuse Grand Mal and Occasional Grand Mal

Both groups of patients did not show an increase in frequency of total paroxysmal or of any individual paroxysmal potential.

4.1.4. Lennox Syndrome

An increased frequency was observed in atypical sp-w-c and in total sp-w-c.

4.1.5. Absence Petit Mal

A higher frequency was observed in 3/s sp-w-c (20 %, P < 0.001), in atypical sp-w-c (20 %, P < 0.01), in total sp-w-c (40 %, P < 0.001), and in total patients with paroxysmal abnormalities (74 %, P < 0.05).

4.1.6. Myoclonic Petit Mal

There was an increased frequency in 3/s sp-w-c (21 %, P < 0.005), in atypical sp-w-c (26 %, P < 0.005), in total sp-w-c (47 %, P < 0.001), and in patients with total paroxysmal patterns (84 %, P < 0.025).

4.1.7. Total Petit Mal

Increased frequencies were observed in 3/s sp-w-c (17 %, P < 0.001), in atypical sp-w-c (26 %, P < 0.001), in total sp-w-c (43 %, P < 0.001), and in patients with total paroxysmal patterns (78 %, P < 0.001).

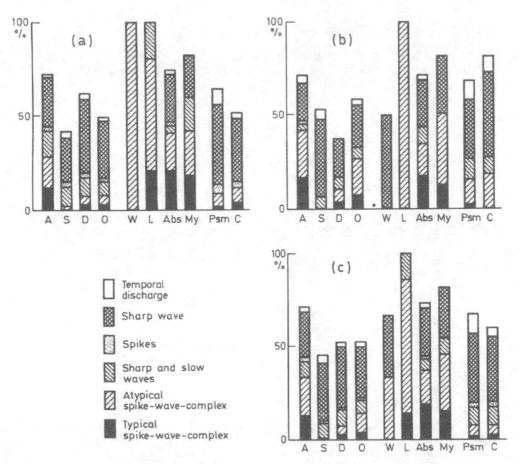

Fig. 3a-c. Type of seizure and paroxysmal EEG abnormalities. (a) Male patients. (b) Female patients. (c) Total patients

4.1.8. Psychomotor Epilepsy

A lower frequency was found in atypical sp-w-c (1.5 %, P < 0.05) and in patients with total sp-w-c (1.5 %, P < 0.01). On the other hand, the frequency in temporal discharge (9 %, P < 0.01) was increased.

4.1.9. Cortical Epilepsy

No significant difference was found.

4.2. Female Patients (Table 15, Figure 3b)

4.2.1. Awakening Grand Mal

There was a higher frequency in 3/s sp-w-c (16 %, P < 0.001), in atypical sp-w-c (25 %, P < 0.05), and in patients with total sp-w-c (41 %, P < 0.001).

4.2.2. Grand Mal During Sleep

Typical or atypical sp-w-c was not found in patients with grand mal during sleep.

4.2.3. Diffuse Grand Mal

The frequency of total patients with paroxysmal abnormalities was decreased (38 %, P < 0.01).

4.2.4. Absence Petit Mal

There was an increased frequency in 3/s sp-w-c (17 %, P < 0.01).

4.2.5. Myoclonic Petit Mal

A higher frequency was seen in atypical sp-w-c (13 %, P < 0.05) and in patients with total sp-w-c (50 %, P < 0.01).

4.2.6. Total Petit Mal

The frequency observed was increased in 3/s sp-w-c (15 %, P < 0.01), in atypical sp-w-c (25 %, P < 0.05), in total sp-w-c (40 %, P < 0.001), and in patients with total paroxysmal EEG (77 %, P < 0.05).

4.2.7. Occasional Grand Mal, Psychomotor Epilepsy, and Cortical Epilepsy

There was no obvious relation among these types of seizure and EEG abnormality. A higher frequency was only observed in temporal discharge in patients with psychomotor epilepsy (11 %, P < 0.05).

4.3. Total Patients (Figure 3c)

4.3.1. Awakening Grand Mal

There was an increased frequency in 3/s sp-w-c (13 %, P < 0.001), in atypical sp-w-c (20 %, P < 0.001), in total sp-w-c (33 %, P < 0.001), and in total patients with paroxysmal patterns (71 %, P < 0.001).

4.3.2. Grand Mal During Sleep

A decreased frequency was found in 3/s sp-w-c (no patient), in atypical sp-w-c (1.1 %, P < 0.01), in total sp-w-c (1.1 %, P < 0.001), and in total patients with paroxysmal patterns (46 %, P < 0.01).

4.3.3. Diffuse Grand Mal

A decreased frequency was observed in patients with total sp-w-c (52 %, P < 0.05).

4.3.4. Occasional Grand Mal

No significant difference was revealed.

4.3.5. West Syndrome

About 67 % of patients showed paroxysmal EEG abnormalities.

4.3.6. Lennox Syndrome

There was an increased frequency of atypical sp-w-c (60 %, P < 0.01) and in patients with total sp-w-c (60 %, P < 0.05).

4.3.7. Absence Petit Mal

There was an increased frequency of 3/s sp-w-c (19 %, P < 0.001), of atypical sp-w-c (19 %, P < 0.05), of total sp-w-c (37 %, P < 0.001), and in total patients with paroxysmal patterns (73 %, P < 0.05).

4.3.8. Myoclonic Petit Mal

An increased frequency was found in 3/s sp-w-c (17 %, P < 0.001), in atypical sp-w-c (31 %, P < 0.001), in total sp-w-c (49 %, P < 0.001), and in total patients with paroxysmal patterns (83 %, P < 0.01).

4.3.9. Total Petit Mal

An increased frequency was observed in 3/s sp-w-c (16 %, P < 0.001), in atypical sp-w-c (26 %, P < 0.001), in total sp-w-c (42 %, P < 0.001), and in total patients with paroxysmal patterns (77 %, P < 0.001).

4.3.10. Psychomotor Epilepsy

A lower frequency was found in atypical sp-w-c (5.9 %, P < 0.05) and in total sp-w-c (7.6 %, P < 0.01); however, the frequency of temporal discharge was increased (10 %, P < 0.001).

4.3.11. Cortical Epilepsy

No significant difference was observed.

4.4. Discussion of Correlation Between Type of Seizure and Paroxysmal EEG Abnormalities

The incidence of paroxysmal or nonparoxysmal EEG abnormalities in patients with each type of seizure has been reported by various authors. As stated previously, results are influenced by many factors, mainly the sampling methods used, age and sex of patients, diagnostic criteria, and methods of EEG examination.

CHRISTIAN (1968) reported EEG abnormality in about 75 % adult epileptics. Among children, the incidence of EEG abnormality is reported to be increased to 92 % (MATTHES, 1961). The frequency in the present study was 59 %.

According to AJMONE MARSAN and ZIVIN (1970), the number of patients with positive EEG findings rose from 56 % at the first examination to 83 % at repeated examinations. They used in their study such effective methods of provocation as hyperventilation, photic stimulation, drugs, sleep induction, etc.

4.4.1. Awakening Grand Mal

GÄNSHIRT and VETTER (1961) observed more than 41 % of patients with 3-4/s sp-w-c and CHRISTIAN (1960, 1961) observed 41 %. FURUICHI (1969) reported 50 % of patients with EEG abnormality, including 45 % with bilateral paroxysmal activity and 33 % with sp-w-c. BEYER and JOVANOVIC (1966) reported 68 % of patients exhibiting seizure potential, including 29 % with 3/s sp-w-c, 7.5 % with atypical sp-w-c, and 14 % with focal abnormality. KRISCHEK (1962) found that 46 % of patients had EEG abnormalities. As far as the present authors are aware, there are not data reported concerning children. In the authors' study, 33 % of the

total patients exhibited sp-w-c and 71 % exhibited paroxysmal
EEG abnormalities. These results were similar to those found in
previous studies mentioned above. An increase in the frequency
of typical, atypical, and total sp-w-c, as well as of total paroxysmal EEG abnormalities in patients with awakening grand mal
was found in the present study. These are all characteristic
findings for awakening grand mal.

4.4.2. Grand Mal During Sleep

CHRISTIAN (1960, 1961) found 40 % of patients with EEG abnormality, including only 3 % with 3-4/s sp-w-c. The incidence of total
dysrhythmia and paroxysmal dysrhythmia was lower (17 % and 10 %,
respectively) than in patients with awakening grand mal (63 %
and 48 %). GÄNSHIRT and VETTER (1961) found 3 % of patients had
seizure potentials at rest, with the frequency increasing to
12.5 % during hyperventilation and 63 % during sleep. Sleep provocation was very effective in patients with S-GM. FURUICHI
(1969) showed that 60 % of patients exhibited an EEG abnormality,
including 19 % with sp-w-c, 26 % with bilateral paroxysmal activity, and a high frequency of patients (39 %) with total abnormality, mainly in the mid-temporal area (15 %). KRISCHEK (1962)
reported EEG abnormalities in 18.8 % of patients. KRUSE (1964)
found seizure potentials among 76 % of children studied. The
difference of incidence of EEG abnormalities between children
and adults may be influenced by age and pathogenesis (GÄNSHIRT
and VETTER, 1961).

CHRISTIAN (1961) studied 150 patients with grand mal during
sleep and a similar number with awakening grand mal. In the
former group he found a statistically higher incidence of normal
EEG patterns, temporal sharp wave, focal abnormalities, and
sleep provocation rate. The patients with grand mal during sleep
also had a lower incidence of abnormal background, diffuse dysrhythmia, paroxysmal dysrhythmia, 3-4/s as well as total sp-w-c,
and pathologic changes during hyperventilation, especially seizure potentials. In another study of 150 patients, each with
grand mal during sleep associated with petit mal, and in patients with awakening grand mal also associated with petit mal,
CHRISTIAN (1960) found a similar difference in EEG patterns.
In this study, when petit mal was associated with grand mal
during sleep, a higher incidence of background abnormality, diffuse dysrhythmia, slow sharp wave, and seizure potentials during
hyperventilation were observed. When awakening grand mal was
associated with petit mal, a significant increase was noted in
paroxysmal dysrhythmia, 3-4/s sp-w-c, and general changes during
hyperventilation. The only common finding was a decrease of normal EEG in both groups.

The observed effect was different in the EEG caused by association
with petit mal in patients with awakening grand mal and in those
with grand mal during sleep.

In the present study and for those patients with S-GM, a decrease
in frequencies in typical, atypical, and total sp-w-c, and total

paroxysmal EEG abnormalities was found. The frequency of paroxysmal EEG abnormalities of 46 % and that of total sp-w-c of 1.1 %
in the present study corresponds with the previous reports cited
above.

4.4.3. Diffuse Grand Mal

With respect to the type of seizure, the frequency of EEG abnormality in this study was highest in patients with A-GM, lowest
in those with S-GM, and intermediate in those with D-GM. These
data agree with previously reported studies (CHRISTIAN, 1961;
KRISCHEK, 1962; FURUICHI, 1969).

4.4.4. West Syndrome

In our study, no definite conclusion could be drawn, since only
a small number of patients were at our disposal. Previously reported studies of patients with West syndrome indicate the characteristic EEG abnormality as hypsarrhythmia (GIBBS and GIBBS,
1952, among others). The incidence of EEG abnormality has been
reported to be between 50 % (BOWERS and JEAVONE, 1959) and 100 %
(GASTAUT et al., 1964).

4.4.5. Lennox Syndrome

Among patients with Lennox syndrome, 2-2.5/s slow sp-w-c was
most frequently observed (SCHNEIDER et al., 1970, 25 %; OHTAHARA
et al., 1970, 32.5 %; KRUSE, 1968, 67 %). These findings correspond with those revealed in the present study. The incidence
of hypsarrhythmia was the second most frequent abnormality; however, the incidence was less frequent than that found in patients
with West syndrome (25 %: SCHNEIDER et al., 1970; 26 %: KARBOWSKI
et al., 1970).

4.4.6. Absence Petit Mal

The characteristic EEG of 3/s sp-w-c was most common among patients with absence petit mal, with an incidence between 60 and
80 % (JASPER and KERSCHMAN, 1941; GIBBS et al., 1943; HOLOWACH
et al., 1962; GIBBERD, 1966). On the other hand, the type of
seizure among patients with 3/s sp-w-c was predominantly pyknoleptic petit mal or absence petit mal (DALBY, 1969, 47 %; GOTO,
1957, 82 %). An increased frequency of 3/s sp-w-c was reported
among patients with petit mal compared to those with grand mal
(CLARK and KNOTT, 1955; LUNDERVOLD et al., 1959). A higher incidence of petit mal than of grand mal was also found among patients with 3/s sp-w-c. As shown in the present study, patients
with absence PM had an increased frequency not only of typical
sp-w-c but also of atypical and total sp-w-c. Close correlation

between certain types of seizures and typical sp-w-c was found
not only in absence petit mal but also to a lesser degree among
patients with awakening grand mal. These electro-clinical associations will be discussed later in this chapter.

4.4.7. Myoclonic Petit Mal

JANZ and CHRISTIAN (1957) found EEG abnormalities, including
multiple sp-w-c, in 92 % of patients during repeated examinations
using various activation methods. HORI (1959) found many patients
with myoclonic epilepsy among patients with multiple sp-w-c.
Among children AICARDI and CHEVRIE (1971) observed 3/s irregular
sp-w-c in long duration. The present study revealed a correlation
similar to that found in patients with absence petit mal and in
those with myoclonic petit mal. However, there was a slight difference: the correlation observed was less noticable in typical
sp-w-c, but was more marked in atypical sp-w-c in the case of
myoclonic petit mal. This will be discussed in Chapter V.

4.4.8. Psychomotor Epilepsy

A relatively low incidence of EEG abnormalities was found by
JASPER et al. (1951), GASTAUT (1954), AJMONE MARSAN and RALSTON
(1957), von HEDENSTRÖM and SCHORSCH (1958), and MATTHES (1961),
among others. CHRISTIAN (1968) reported bilateral synchronous
sp-w-c in 6 % only, but a high incidence of 4-6/s sharp waves
or sharp and slow waves, as did MEYER-MICKELEIT (1953). JASPER
et al. (1951) and GASTAUT (1950) found more sharp waves (52 %
and 75 %, respectively) than spike activity (37 % and 43 %,
respectively). CHRISTIAN (1962) found a rather high frequency
of EEG abnormalities (85 %, dysrhythmia and background abnormality), including 70 % of focal abnormality mainly in the temporal
area. He also found a higher frequency of bilateral focal abnormality in patients with idiopathic epilepsy than in those
with unilateral focal abnormality. Conversely, in patients with
symptomatic psychomotor seizure, he found a higher frequency of
unilateral focal abnormality.

GLASER and GOLUB (1955) observed EEG abnormalities in 66 % of
110 psychomotor epileptic children. EEG examination showed (1)
relatively infrequent focal temporal discharge, (2) a slight increase of abnormality during sleep (a difference may exist between adults and children), (3) a rather high frequency of bilateral synchronous 3/s sp-w-c (13 %) as well as atypical 1.5-3/s
sp-w-c (18 %), and (4) during sleep, bitemporal spikes were more
frequent than unilateral temporal focus. On the other hand, JERAS
(1960) observed temporal foci in 84 % of 50 child patients.
NIEDERMEYER (1957) also found a high frequency, 81 %, of EEG
abnormalities in children. Of 47 patients, 21 showed focal abnormality (45 %); temporal focus was found in 18 (38 %). HESS
and NEUHAUS (1952) studied 106 children, 81 % of whom showed
abnormal EEG including 62 % with focal abnormality. GLASER and
GOLUB (1955) indicated that if patients also suffered from petit

mal, all of them (10 patients) revealed bilateral synchronous
3/s sp-w-c. However, if they did not suffer from petit mal, most
of the patients showed atypical sp-w-c (20 of 24 patients). The
difference was statistically significant (P(Fisher) = 0.000008).
Some authors observed 3/s sp-w-c (MAGNUS et al., 1952; FUSTER
et al., 1954; NIEDERMEYER, 1954; CHRISTIAN, 1955; GLASER and
GOLUB, 1955; GARSCHE, 1956; JUNG, 1957; MATTHES, 1961).

Such a relatively wide variety, not only in the frequency of EEG
abnormalities but also in their nature and localization, suggest
a heterogeneity in the pathogenesis of this type of seizure.

4.4.9. Cortical Epilepsy

In the present study, paroxysmal EEG abnormalities were found in
60 % of patients. Only 3 patients were observed with sp-w-c
(7.5 %). These frequencies did not differ from those found in
the total patients. The highest frequency of focal abnormality
was found in patients who suffered from cortical epilepsy (33 %,
P < 0.001). KRUSE (1964) observed 88 % of seizure potentials
among children, GIBBS and GIBBS (1952) 84 %, whereas JANZ (1969)
reported only 22 % among adults. This relatively large difference
seems to depend on differences in the age and pathogenesis of
the patients studied.

4.4.10. Idiopathic and Symptomatic Epilepsy

ROBINSON and OSTERHELD (1947) found a higher frequency of EEG
abnormality in patients with idiopathic epilepsy than in patients
with symptomatic epilepsy (91 % : 60 %, P < 0.001, calculated
by the authors); however, there was no difference in the frequency of sp-w-c (27 % vs. 22 %). In the authors' study, sp-w-c
EEG was found in 16 % of the total patients; the frequency increased in patients with a familial predisposition to the disease
(35 % vs. 14 %, P < 0.001), but decreased in patients with exogenous factors (12 % vs. 18 %, not significant); it was not
common in patients with cortical epilepsy.

4.5. Comparison of Findings Between Male and Female Patients

As described in Chapter III.4, male and female patients revealed
a relatively similar correlation between type of seizure and
paroxysmal EEG abnormalities.

5. Coefficient of Contingency Analysis of Correlation Between Type of Seizure and Paroxysmal EEG Abnormalities

As already described, patients with certain types of seizures
showed a statistically significant increase in paroxysmal as

well as sp-w-c EEG. A significant correlation between type of
seizure and paroxysmal EEG abnormalities was found.

With regard to this correlation, the authors made the following
analysis. The observed x^2 value was used to calculate a coefficient of contingency (c_1) by the following formula:

$$c_1 = \sqrt{\frac{x^2}{N + x^2}}$$

N = number of total patients studied.

Depending upon a higher or lower frequency observed, c_1 has either
a plus or minus value. With respect to an increase or decrease in
the observed distribution, the most extreme example (the greatest
increase or decrease) was estimated and the maximum or minimum
coefficient of contingency was calculated (c_2). The relative coefficient of contingency was considered to be $c_r = c_1/c_2$; therefore this value varies between -1.00 and +1.00. The value of the
relative coefficient of contingency (c_r) in various correlations
has been indicated (Table 16).

A marked positive association (a high positive value of the relative coefficient of contingency ($c_r > 0.5$)) was found between:

1. <u>Awakening grand mal</u> and 3/s sp-w-c, atypical sp-w-c, total
   sp-w-c, irregular sp-w-c, 2-2.5/s sp-w-c, 3.5-5/s sp-w-c, and
   multiple sp-w-c.

2. <u>Lennox syndrome</u> and atypical sp-w-c, total sp-w-c, and total
   paroxysmal abnormality.

3. <u>Absence petit mal</u> and 3/s sp-w-c, total sp-w-c, and multiple
   sp-w-c.

4. <u>Myoclonic petit mal</u> and total sp-w-c and total paroxysmal
   abnormality.

5. <u>Total petit mal</u> and 3/s sp-w-c, atypical sp-w-c, irregular
   sp-w-c, 2-2.5/s sp-w-c, 3.5-5/s sp-w-c, and multiple sp-w-c.

6. <u>Psychomotor epilepsy</u> and temporal discharge.

7. <u>Cortical epilepsy</u> showed no positive association.

A marked negative association which had a high negative value of
the relative coefficient of contingency ($c_r < -0.5$) was found
between:

1. <u>Grand mal during sleep</u> and 3/s sp-w-c, atypical sp-w-c,
   irregular sp-w-c, multiple sp-w-c, and total sp-w-c.

2. <u>Diffuse grand mal</u> and total sp-w-c.

3. <u>Lennox syndrome</u> and temporal discharge.

4. <u>Myoclonic PM</u> and temporal discharge.

5. <u>Psychomotor epilepsy</u> and atypical sp-w-c, 3.5-5/s sp-w-c,
   multiple sp-w-c, and total sp-w-c.

6. <u>Cortical epilepsy</u> showed no negative correlation.

These correlations are illustrated in Figure 4a.

28

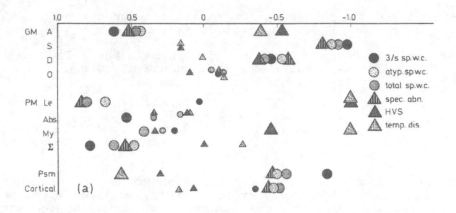

Fig. 4a. Relative coefficient of contingency on type of seizure and paroxysmal EEG abnormalities

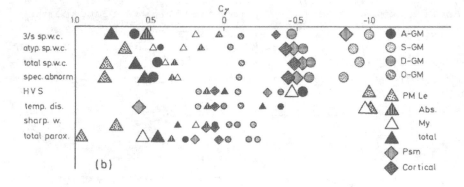

Fig. 4b. Relative coefficient of contingency on paroxysmal EEG abnormalities and type of seizure

The most evident positive associations were observed between patients with awakening grand mal and those with 3/s as well as multiple sp-w-c; patients with absence petit mal and those with 3/s sp-w-c; total patients with petit mal and total patients with sp-w-c; and patients with psychomotor epilepsy and those with temporal discharge.

The most significant negative association was found between sp-w-c and those with grand mal during sleep, diffuse grand mal, and with psychomotor epilepsy.

The correlation could also be analyzed from the standpoint of the EEG pattern, i.e., as a correlation between EEG and type of seizure. The results observed are illustrated in Figure 4b. In Figure 4a and b, the electroclinical correlations are clearly demonstrated.

A positive correlation was found between absence petit mal and 3/s sp-w-c EEG (c_r = +0.647), West syndrome and hypsarrhythmia (c_r = +0.692), cortical seizure and focal EEG abnormality (c_r = +0.537). A negative correlation was found between absence PM and focal EEG abnormality when the results reported by HESS and NEUHAUS (1952) were analyzed.

6. Type of Seizure and Individual Paroxysmal EEG Pattern

Tables 17 and 18 show the correlations between types of seizures and paroxysmal EEG findings in which all potentials were separately counted.

6.1. Male Patients

Correlation in male patients is shown in Table 17.

6.1.1. Awakening Grand Mal

An increased frequency was observed in patients with 3/s sp-w-c (11 %, P < 0.05), in irregular sp-w-c (10 %, P < 0.01), and in those with multiple sp-w-c (12 %, P < 0.01).

6.1.2. Absence Petit Mal

An increased frequency was found in patients with 3/s sp-w-c (20 %, P < 0.001), irregular sp-w-c (14 %, P < 0.01), 2-2.5/s sp-w-c (9 %, P < 0.05), 3.5-5/s sp-w-c (11 %, P < 0.01), and multiple sp-w-c (14 %, P < 0.05).

6.1.3. Myoclonic Petit Mal

An increased frequency of patients with 3/s sp-w-c (21 %, P < 0.01) and irregular sp-w-c (21 %, P < 0.001) was indicated.

6.1.4. Total Petit Mal

The frequency in patients with 3/s sp-w-c (20 %, P < 0.001), irregular sp-w-c (19 %, P < 0.001), and multiple sp-w-c (12 %, P < 0.001) was increased.

6.1.5. Psychomotor Epilepsy

The frequency of temporal discharge was increased (15 %, $P < 0.001$).

6.1.6. Diffuse Grand Mal, Grand Mal During Sleep and Cortical Epilepsy

No marked difference was observed.

6.2. Female Patients

The correlation in female patients is shown in Table 18.

6.2.1. Awakening Grand Mal

There was an increased frequency of patients with 3/s sp-w-c (16 %, $P < 0.001$), 3.5-5/s sp-w-c (18 %, $P < 0.01$), and multiple sp-w-c (22 %, $P < 0.001$).

6.2.2. Grand Mal During Sleep and Diffuse Grand Mal

A decreased frequency was found in 3.5-5/s sp-w-c as well as in multiple sp-w-c ($P < 0.01$, $P < 0.05$, respectively).

6.2.3. Absence Petit Mal

The frequency of 3/s sp-w-c as well as multiple sp-w-c was increased (17 %, $P < 0.01$, and 23 %, $P < 0.01$, respectively).

6.2.4. Total Petit Mal

An increased frequency was observed in patients with 3/s sp-w-c (15 %, $P < 0,01$), 3.5-5/s sp-w-c (6 %, $P < 0.05$), and multiple sp-w-c (21 %, $P < 0.01$).

6.2.5. Psychomotor Epilepsy

The frequency of temporal discharge was increased (13 %, $P < 0.05$). Conversely the frequency of 3.5-5/s sp-w-c was lower ($P < 0.05$).

6.2.6. Psychomotor Epilepsy and Cortical Epilepsy

There was a decreased frequency of multiple sp-w-c (3.1 %, $P < 0.05$).

6.3. Total Number of Patients

6.3.1. Awakening Grand Mal

There was an increased frequency of 3/s sp-w-c (13 %, P < 0.001), irregular sp-w-c (9 %, P < 0.01), 2-2.5/s sp-w-c (4.8 %, P < 0.05), 3.5-5/s sp-w-c (9.5 %, P < 0.01), and multiple sp-w-c (16 %, P < 0.001).

6.3.2. Grand Mal During Sleep

There were no findings in patients with 3/s sp-w-c, in irregular sp-w-c, and in those with multiple sp-w-c.

6.3.3. Absence Petit Mal

There was an increased frequency of patients with 3/s sp-w-c (19 %, P < 0.001), in irregular sp-w-c (10 %, P < 0.05), 3.5-5/s sp-w-c (11 %, P < 0.05), and in those with multiple sp-w-c (19 %, P < 0.001).

6.3.4. Myoclonic Petit Mal

The frequency of 3/s sp-w-c was higher (17 %, P < 0.01).

6.3.5. Total Petit Mal

The frequency observed was higher in patients with 3/s sp-w-c (18 %, P < 0.001), in irregular sp-w-c (12 %, P < 0.001), in 2-2.5/s sp-w-c (6.6 %, P < 0.01), in 3.5-5/s sp-w-c (12 %, P < 0.001), and in those with multiple sp-w-c (20 %, P < 0.001).

6.3.6. Psychomotor Epilepsy

There was a decreased frequency of patients with 3.5-5/s sp-w-c (0.8 %, P < 0.05) and in multiple sp-w-c (1.7 %, P < 0.01). Conversely, the frequency of patients with temporal discharge was higher (14 %, P < 0.001).

6.3.7. Diffuse Grand Mal, Occasional Grand Mal, Lennox Syndrome, Cortical Epilepsy

No marked difference was observed.

7. Type of Seizure and EEG Diagnosis

In this section the nonspecific abnormal, epileptic abnormal, and focal abnormalities of EEG patterns are discussed (see Table 19, EEG diagnosis).

7.1. Male Patients (Table 19)

The frequency of abnormal EEG (c+d+e under EEG diagnosis in Table 19) was higher in patients with A-GM (54 %, P < 0.05), myoclonic PM (71 %, P < 0.05), total PM (65 %, P < 0.001), and psychomotor epilepsy (55 %, P < 0.05). EEG abnormalities characteristic of epilepsy (see d under EEG diagnosis in Table 19) were higher in patients with A-GM (27 %, P < 0.001), Lennox syndrome (100 %, P < 0.001), absence PM (37 %, P < 0.001), and total PM (41 %, P < 0.001). Conversely, EEG abnormalities were decreased in patients with S-GM, D-GM, and with psychomotor epilepsy (1.5 %, P < 0.01).

The focal abnormality was increased in patients with cortical epilepsy (31 %), D-GM (20 %) and with psychomotor epilepsy (31 %, P < 0.001), while it was lower in patients with A-GM (6 %, P < 0.01) and absence PM (5.7 %).

7.2. Female Patients (Table 20)

The frequency of abnormal EEG (EEG diagnosis, c+d+e, Table 20) in patients with D-GM was found to be lower (31 %, P < 0.05). The epileptic abnormal EEG was higher in patients with A-GM (41 %, P < 0.001), absence PM (40 %, P < 0.01), myoclonic PM (50 %, P < 0.01), and total PM (44 %, P < 0.001). However, it was lower in patients with S-GM (2.8 %, P < 0.01) and D-GM (6.3 %, P < 0.05).

The focal abnormality was higher in patients with cortical epilepsy (36 %, P < 0.05) and S-GM, but lower in patients with total PM (1.9 %, P < 0.05), A-GM, absence, and with myoclonic PM.

7.3. Total Number of Patients

There was an increased frequency of abnormal EEG (c+d+e) in patients with A-GM (54 %, P < 0.01), Lennox syndrome (P(Fisher) = 0.0033), myoclonic PM (64 %, P < 0.05), total PM (60 %, P < 0.001), and psychomotor epilepsy (54 %, P < 0.05). A lower frequency was found in total patients with S-GM and D-GM (36 %, P < 0.01).

The abnormal EEG characteristic of epilepsy was more common in patients with A-GM (33 %, P < 0.001), absence PM (39 %, P < 0.001), myoclonic PM (42 %, P < 0.001), and total PM (42 %, P < 0.001). It was found less often in patients with S-GM (4.5 %, P < 0.01),

D-GM (6.1 %, P < 0.01), psychomotor epilepsy (5.9 %, P < 0.01), and was not significant in cortical epilepsy.

The focal abnormality was most common in patients with cortical epilepsy (33 %, P < 0.001) and in those with psychomotor epilepsy (27 %, P < 0.001); however, it was decreased in patients with A-GM (5.4 %, P < 0.001), in absence PM (4.3 %, P < 0.05), and in those with total PM (5.7 %, P < 0.01).

7.4. Comparison Between Frequencies of EEG Abnormalities in Male and Female Patients

A similar distribution of frequency of EEG abnormalities in male and female patients has been shown; it was increased in frequency in patients with A-GM, Lennox syndrome, absence PM, myoclonic PM, total PM, psychomotor, and in those with cortical epilepsy. Conversely, a decreased frequency was found in patients with S-GM, D-GM, and with O-GM.

8. Comparison Between Correlation Found in Male and Female Patients

As indicated above, marked similar correlations between type of seizure and paroxysmal EEG patterns were found in both male and female patients.

9. Type of Seizure and Basic EEG Rhythm (Tables 19 and 20)

9.1. α-EEG

The total number of patients with A-GM showed a higher incidence of high voltage α-activity (14 % or 21 of 147 patients, P < 0.05) than did patients with other types of seizure; however, a lower incidence of high voltage α-activity was found in the total number of patients with S-GM and D-GM (6.4 % or 11 of 171 patients, P < 0.05) than in patients with other types of seizure. Patients with absence and myoclonic PM, and Lennox syndrome showed an increased incidence of high voltage α-activity, but no patient with cortical epilepsy showed high voltage α-activity (P(Fisher) = 0.012).

These findings were observed in both male and in female patients; the differences, however, were not statistically significant. An increased incidence of high voltage α-activity and a decreased incidence of normal α-activity was observed in female patients compared with males (15 % vs. 6.9 %, P < 0.01, and 72 % vs. 84 %, P < 0.01, respectively).

In previous studies, JAVANOVIC (1967) found some differences concerning frequency and amplitude of α-rhythm among patients with some types of grand mal. Patients with awakening grand mal had the lowest frequency and the highest amplitude (8.3/s, 110 µV); those with grand mal during sleep showed the highest frequency and the lowest amplitude (10/s, 60 µV); patients with diffuse grand mal were intermediate (9/s, 100 µV).

9.2. β-EEG

9.2.1. Male Patients

The incidence of β-EEG was lower in total patients with S-GM and D-GM (8 %, P < 0.01), but higher in patients with myoclonic PM (35 %, P < 0.01).

9.2.2. Female Patients

An increased frequency of β-EEG was found in patients with myoclonic PM (50 %, P < 0.01) and with total PM (35 %, P < 0.05).

9.2.3. Total Number of Patients

The frequency of β-EEG was higher in patients with myoclonic PM (42 %, P < 0.001) and with total PM (26 %, P < 0.01); however, it decreased in patients with S-GM (10 %, P < 0.05). A higher incidence of β-EEG was observed in patients with absence PM, A-GM, and with cortical epilepsy, and a lower frequency was found in those with D-GM. However, the difference was not statistically significant. A higher incidence of β-EEG among epileptic patients (8.5 % for males, 13 % for females) than among the general population (5.5 % for males, 12 % for females) was reported by VOGEL and GÖTZE (1962); the difference was statistically significant for males only (P < 0.05). In previous analyses, no correlation was undertaken.

9.2.4. Comparison Between Frequencies of β-EEG in Male and Female Patients

A similar analysis of the frequency of occurrence of the β-EEG in various types of seizure in male and in female patients found a higher frequency in patients with myoclonic PM, total PM, A-GM, and in those with cortical epilepsy, and a lower frequency in patients with S-GM, D-GM, and with Lennox syndrome. Differences were observed in patients with absence PM as well as psychomotor epilepsy.

The difference between the frequency of occurrence of β-EEG in male and in female patients was significant (23 % vs. 9 %, P < 0.05).

9.3. Slow Waves

In the authors' study slow wave dominant basic rhythm was considered as slow wave EEG. A lower incidence of θ- and δ-waves
was more common in patients with A-GM, myoclonic PM, and with
cortical epilepsy; however, the difference was not statistically
significant. Correlation between type of seizure and incidence
of slow waves is indicated in Tables 19 and 20.

In general, the incidence of slow waves is related to the age
of the patient, as shown by PETERSEN and EEG OLOFSSON (1971) in
their follow-up study of normal children aged 1 - 15. A high incidence of slow waves was observed in patients with West syndrome
and Lennox syndrome involving mainly young children. Epileptic
children were apt to show more slow waves than adult epileptics
despite the same type of seizure, i.e., in patients with grand
mal during sleep, psychomotor, and with cortical epilepsy (see
LENNOX and DAVIS, 1950; JERAS, 1970; MATTHES, 1961).

9.4. Low Voltage EEG

An increased incidence of low voltage EEG was found in all patients with occasional grand mal (11 %, P < 0.001); in male patients (11 %, P < 0.01); and in female patients (10 %, P < 0.05).
A decreased frequency of low voltage EEG was found in patients
with A-GM (only one patient P(Fisher) = 0.035). Patients with
Lennox syndrome and with absence PM showed a lower incidence.
The incidence in patients with cortical epilepsy was higher but
the difference was not statistically significant. In some neurologic diseases, an increase of low voltage EEG has been suspected,
e.g., in patients with Huntington's chorea (VOGEL et al., 1961a)
and in those with head trauma (GÖTZE, 1957). ADAM (1959) reported
a negative correlation between low voltage EEG and epilepsy.
Among 665 epileptics, he failed to find any patients with low
voltage EEG. VOGEL (1962) found that patients with and without
this kind of EEG appeared to have the similar incidence of seizure occurrence. Our present study confirmed the findings reported by PINE and PINE (1953) cited by VOGEL and GÖTZE (1959),
that this type of EEG is found in the range of 3 % in normal population.

9.5. Pathologic Findings During Hyperventilation

9.5.1. Male Patients

There was an increased frequency of pathologic findings during
hyperventilation in patients with A-GM (42 %, P < 0.01), absence
PM (54 %, P < 0.001), and myoclonic PM (59 %, P < 0.01). The
frequency in patients with S-GM was lower (13 %, P < 0.01).

9.5.2. Female Patients

An increased frequency of pathologic findings during hyperventilation was found in patients with A-GM (43 %, P < 0.05), absence PM (49 %, P < 0.05), and myoclonic PM (56 %, P < 0.05). The frequency was lower in patients with S-GM (8 %, P < 0.01) and in patients with psychomotor epilepsy (19 %, P < 0.05).

9.5.3. Total Patients

An increased frequency was observed in patients with A-GM (42 %, P < 0.001), absence PM (51 %, P < 0.001), and myoclonic PM (58 %, P < 0.001). The frequency was lower in patients with S-GM (11 %, P < 0.001) and in those with psychomotor epilepsy (20 %, P < 0.01).

Apparently the type of seizure and age of patients are the determining factors as to the effect of hyperventilation. There was a marked difference in effectiveness between patients with awakening grand mal and those with grand mal during sleep.

With sleep activation, GÄNSHIRT (1961) and CHRISTIAN (1968) found a high frequency of pathologic EEG, including 3-3.5/s sp-w-c in patients with awakening grand mal. Sleep activation was more effective in patients with grand mal during sleep than in those with awakening grand mal, as indicated by GÄNSHIRT and CHRISTIAN. This method was also effective in patients with psychomotor epilepsy; 90 % of the patients were found to have temporal foci compared with only 30 % at routine examination (CHRISTIAN, 1968).

GABOR and AJMONE MARSAN (1969) observed a higher frequency of nonparoxysmal abnormalities during hyperventilation in patients with focal or bilateral synchronous epileptic discharge (71 %) than in those without bilateral involvement (30 %); the difference was statistically significant according to our calculations.

9.5.4. Comparison Between Frequencies of Pathologic Findings During Hyperventilation in Male and Female Patients

A similar tendency was found in the reaction during hyperventilation in male and female patients, as shown in Tables 19 and 20.

9.6. Focal Sign

9.6.1. Male Patients (Table 19)

A lower frequency of focal sign was found in patients with A-GM (7 %, P < 0.001); however, the frequency was higher in patients with psychomotor epilepsy (31 %, P < 0.001), as well as in those with cortical epilepsy (31 %, P < 0.05).

9.6.2. Female Patients (Table 20)

There was a decreased frequency of focal sign in patients with A-GM (6 %, P < 0.05) and in total PM (4 %, P < 0.05); conversely, the frequency in patients with psychomotor epilepsy was higher (30 %, P < 0.001) as it was in those with cortical epilepsy (36 %).

9.6.3. Total Number of Patients

There was a higher frequency of focal sign in patients with psychomotor epilepsy (30 %, P < 0.001) and with cortical epilepsy (33 %, P < 0.01); however, there was a lower incidence in A-GM (7 %, P < 0.001), in absence PM (6 %, P < 0.05), and in total PM (7.5 %, P < 0.05). These findings correspond with those published in previous studies. Focal sign was frequently observed in patients with Lennox syndrome (KRUSE, 1968), in psychomotor epilepsy (NIEDERMEYER, 1957), and in those with cortical epilepsy (KRUSE, 1964). A low frequency of focal sign was found in patients with absence PM (JANZ, 1955; CALDERON and PAAL, 1957; BAMBERGER and MATTHES, 1959), myoclonic petit mal (JANZ and CHRISTIAN, 1957) and awakening grand mal (CHRISTIAN, 1960, 1961; KRISCHEK, 1962).

With the same type of seizure, children seemed to show more focal abnormality than adults with respect to grand mal during sleep: 71 % in children (KRUSE, 1964) and 12.5 % in adults (CHRISTIAN, 1968); and with respect to cortical epilepsy: 96 % in children (KRUSE, 1964) and 52 % in adults (LUNDERVOLD et al., 1959). The opposite was found in psychomotor epilepsy: 23 % in children (JERAS, 1970) and 76 % in adults (MEYER-MICKELEIT, 1953). With respect to the influence of age at onset of seizure, the authors' data show an increase of focal abnormality in (1) younger female patients between 10 and 34 years (9 %, P < 0.05); (2) early-onset male patients as well as females aged 0 - 1 year (29 % and 33 %, respectively); (3) late-onset female patients over 35 years (30 %, P < 0.05), and (4) in the total number of patients aged 35 - 39 years (32 %, P < 0.05).

CALDERON and PAAL (1957) and O'BRIEN et al. (1959) reported a relatively high incidence of focal abnormality in patients with absence petit mal.

9.6.4. Comparison Between Frequencies of Focal EEG Abnormality in Male and Female Patients

A similar distribution of frequency of focal sign in male and female patients with various types of seizures was observed. Common features were an increase of focal sign in patients with S-GM, D-GM, psychomotor, and with cortical epilepsy; and a decrease in patients with A-GM, Lennox syndrome, absence PM, myoclonic PM, and in total patients with PM.

10. Type of Seizure and Familial Predisposition (Tables 19 and 20)

10.1. Male Patients

The frequency of familial predisposition to epilepsy was higher in patients with absence PM (26 %, P < 0.01) and in total PM (20 %, P < 0.05).

10.2. Female Patients

Familial predisposition to epilepsy was found more frequently in patients with absence PM (17 %, P < 0.05) and with total PM (15 %, P < 0.05). However, the number was decreased in the total number of S-GM and D-GM (1.5 %, P < 0.05).

10.3. Total Patients

An increased frequency of familial predisposition to epilepsy was found in patients with absence PM (21 %, P < 0.001) and in patients with total PM (18 %, P < 0.01).

As previously mentioned, the incidence of familial predisposition to epilepsy among patients with specific types of epileptic disease can only be accurately assessed in studies where the number of family members screened or the types of relationships included are clearly defined.

Data pertaining to various types of seizure are summarized in Table 21. The median incidence was higher in West and Lennox syndromes, and in absence PM and in myoclonic petit mal, whereas the figures for grand mal and for cortical epilepsy were lower. These results might be related not only to the type of seizure but also to the age of patients and their age at onset of seizure as discussed in Chapter IV.

10.4. Comparison Between Frequencies of Familial Predisposition to Epilepsy in Male and Female Patients

Common features in male and female patients were an increased frequency of familial predisposition to epilepsy in patients with A-GM, absence PM, myoclonic PM, and in those with total PM; and a decreased frequency in patients with S-GM, O-GM, psychomotor epilepsy, and with cortical epilepsy.

11. Type of Seizure and Exogenous Factors (Tables 19 and 20)

Perinatal and postnatal brain damages such as birth injury, cerebral infection, head trauma, etc., are considered as exogenous factors in this monograph.

11.1. Male Patients

A decreased frequency in the relationship of exogenous factors
was found in patients with A-GM (8.3 %, P < 0.01) and in patients
with absence PM (2.9 %, P < 0.05); conversely, in patients with
cortical epilepsy an increased relationship to exogenous factors
was found (35 %, P < 0.05).

11.2. Female Patients

There was an increased relationship to exogenous factors in patients with cortical epilepsy (27 %, P < 0.05).

11.3. Total Patients

A decreased frequency occurred in patients with A-GM (7.5 %,
P < 0.01), with S-GM (6.7 %, P < 0.05), absence PM (2.9 %, P <
0.01),and total PM (6.6 %, P < 0.01). However, the frequency of
exogenous factors in patients with cortical epilepsy was higher
(33 %, P < 0.001). The frequency in patients with D-GM, O-GM,
and Lennox syndrome was higher, and that in patients with myoclonic PM was lower. Differences, however, were not statistically
significant.

The above findings correspond to those observed in previous
studies. Exogenous factors as a cause of epilepsy were frequently
found as follows:

In West syndrome

    1. 43 % (JANZ and AKOS, 1967)
    2. 53 % (CHARLTON and MELLINGER, 1970)
    3. 87 % (STÖGMANN and LORENZONI, 1970)
    4. 95 % (MATTHES and MALLMANN-MÜHLBERGER, 1963)

In Lennox syndrome

    1. 30 % (SCHNEIDER et al., 1970)
    2. 32 % (DOOSE, 1964b)

In grand mal during sleep

    1. 16 % (KRISCHEK, 1962)
    2. 25 % (KRUSE, 1964)

In diffuse grand mal

    1. 53 % (JANZ, 1969)
    2. 65 % (KRISCHEK, 1962)

In pschomotor epilepsy

    1. 23 % (JERAS, 1970)
    2. 79 % (MEYER-MICKELEIT, 1953)

In cortical epilepsy

    1. 80 % (KRUSE, 1964)

Conversely, a low frequency of exogenous factors was seen as follows:

In absence or pyknoleptic PM

1. 5 % (O'BRIEN et al., 1959)
2. 5 % (LIVINGSTON et al., 1965)
3. 11 % (JANZ, 1955)
4. 15 % (GIBBS and GIBBS, 1952)
5. 30 % (PAAL, 1957)
6. 39 % (BAMBERGER and MATTHES, 1959)

In myoclonic petit mal

1. 13 % (head trauma, JANZ and CHRISTIAN, 1957)

In awakening grand mal

1. 8 % (KRISCHEK, 1962)
2. 10 % (JANZ, 1969)

SIMONSON (1951) and KRISCHEK (1959) found a very high incidence of atrophy of the brain (42 % and 43 %, respectively), indicated by pneumoencephalography of patients with cryptogenic epilepsy. In some patients this might be the result of repeated convulsions, as in Lennox syndrome, where organic brain damage is infrequently primary. The presence of exogenous factors among patients with absence petit mal has been believed to be slight (5 % according to O'BRIEN et al. and LIVINGSTON et al. op. cit.). However, other authors have reported a high incidence of the presence of exogenous factors (39 %: BAMBERGER and MATTHES, 1959); pneumo-encephalographic abnormality (48 %: DALBY, 1969); and focal EEG abnormality (52 %: CALDERON and PAAL, 1957).

Absence petit mal might be associated frequently with grand mal during its course as reported by CLARK and KNOTT, 1955; BAMBERGER and MATTHES, 1959; GIBBERD, 1966; and the authors. Therefore, brain atrophy as well as focal abnormality in the EEG might be caused by convulsions.

In general, our study indicates that the influence of exogenous factors is apparently more frequent in children than in adults.

11.4. Comparison Between Frequencies of Occurrence of Exogenous Factors in Male and Female Patients

The total frequency of occurrence of exogenous factors in male patients was higher than in female patients (17 % vs. 6.3 %, P < 0.001).

12. Clinical Association Between Types of Seizures in the Same Patients

Overall, the 466 patients had 1154 clinical types of seizure (648 for males; 506 for females). The clinical association between types of seizures in the same patients (Tables 22 and 23) are analyzed as follows: the expected number of patients with the additional types of seizure was calculated by using the distribution pattern of the total number of types of seizure (irrespective of association with their main clinical types). For example:

1. In the male patients there were 84 instances of A-GM and 35 of absence PM. Of these patients, 22 had A-GM as well as absence PM indicating the existence of an association.

2. In male patients with A-GM, 84 had a total of 139 clinical types of seizures; therefore, 55 of these clinical types were additional.

3. If, using the same data, no tendency exists for certain types of seizure to occur in association in the same individual, the anticipated number of patients with an association of A-GM and absence PM was calculated as follows: Expected number of additional types of seizures =

$$55 \times \frac{\text{number of patients with absence PM}}{\substack{\text{total number of types of seizure minus} \\ \text{patients with A-GM and patients with O-GM}}}$$

$$= 55 \times \frac{35}{384 - 84 - 45} = 7.5$$

4. Based on a comparison between the number of patients observed in the association and the anticipated probabilities, and evaluation was made to determine whether an increase, decrease, or insignificant deviation existed.

5. The coefficient of contingency was calculated by the following formula (previously expressed in this chapter):

$$c_1 = \sqrt{\frac{\chi^2}{N + \chi^2}}$$

The c_1 takes either a plus or minus value depending upon the results observed in (4) with either an increase or a decrease.

6. The maximum or minimum c_2 was calculated using the most extreme case of association. The relative coefficient of contingency is estimated as $c_r = {}^c1/c_2$.

7. The value of c_r lies between -1 and +1 ($-1 < c_r < +1$). The authors considered that if c_r is greater than +0.5, the observed association is significantly increased (positive), and is smaller than -0.5 (negative association). The results of the analysis are shown in Table 24 and illustrated in Figure 5.

As shown in Tables 22 and 23, a similar distribution of additional types of seizures with a marked positive as well as negative correlation was found in male and in female patients. Table 24 shows the relative coefficient of contingency in the total number of patients. Positive correlations existed between: (1) A-GM and absence PM, myoclonic PM, and Lennox syndrome; (2) S-GM and psychomotor epilepsy; (3) D-GM and psychomotor epilepsy; (4) O-GM and psychomotor, and cortical epilepsy. However, in some associations, the correlations were not as close as in others.

Negative correlations were found between: (1) A-GM and S-GM, D-GM, and psychomotor and cortical epilepsy; (2) S-GM and Lennox syndrome, absence PM, myoclonic PM, and cortical epilepsy; (3) D-GM and Lennox syndrome, myoclonic PM, absence PM, and cortical epilepsy; (4) Lennox syndrome and psychomotor epilepsy; (5) absence PM and psychomotor epilepsy, and cortical epilepsy; (6) myoclonic PM and psychomotor epilepsy; (7) psychomotor epilepsy and cortical epilepsy.

These correlations in the total number of patients (similar to those found in male as well as in female patients) are illustrated in Figure 5. One group included patients with A-GM, myoclonic PM, absence PM, and probably also Lennox syndrome. Patients with S-GM comprised the second group and patients with D-GM the third group. Both of these two groups had a negative correlation with the first group. The negative correlation between the second and the third group was indicated. The fourth group, which included patients with psychomotor epilepsy, had a negative correlation with the first group and with cortical epilepsy. The group of patients with psychomotor epilepsy showed a loose correlation with those with either S-GM or D-GM. No type of seizure was found to be positively correlated with focal epilepsy.

Some previous studies containing data on these correlations are as follows:

West Syndrome. A high incidence of association of West syndrome with both grand mal and Lennox syndrome has been observed (JANZ and MATTHES, 1955; DOOSE et al., 1964b; STÖGMANN and LORENZONI, 1970). The associated grand mal usually occurred during sleep (DOOSE et al., 1964 b).

Lennox Syndrome. Lennox syndrome was frequently found to be associated with grand mal (47 - 84 %), atypical absence petit mal (43 - 68 %), and West syndrome (21 - 30 %) (KRUSE, 1966; LANCE, 1969; SCHNEIDER et al., 1970; BUENO et al., 1970; DOOSE et al., 1964b). Very often the associated grand mal occurred during sleep (JANZ and MATTHES, 1955).

In the authors' study, no positive correlation was found between any types of seizures and Lennox syndrome. Because of the small number of patients available for this analysis, no definite conclusions could be drawn.

Absence Petit Mal. Absence petit mal was found to be associated with grand mal in 38 % of patients by CURRIER et al. (1963) and in 69 % of patients by CLARK and KNOTT (1955). Thirteen percent of the patients had myoclonic seizures (GIBBERD, 1966). Eighty-eight percent of associated grand mal was of the awakening type (JANZ, 1955). Transformation from absence PM to grand mal was observed at puberty (GASTAUT, 1954), and the greatest association with grand mal occurred at the age of 12 - 14 years (HERTOFT, 1963)

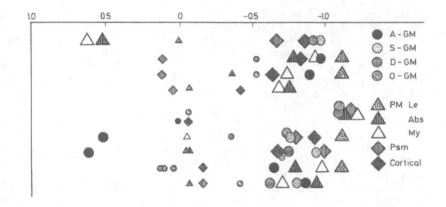

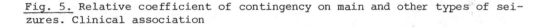

Fig. 5. Relative coefficient of contingency on main and other types of seizures. Clinical association

The incidence of association generally increased with age; 29 %
at age 5, 48 % at 9, and 46 % at 25 years (JANZ, 1969). These
results of seizure appear to indicate that the association rate
depends on age of onset as well as follow-up time. Children
showed a decreased incidence. Petit mal developing into grand
mal was frequently observed whereas the reverse occurred rarely
(HOLOWACH et al., 1962; LIVINGSTON et al., 1965; GIBBERD, 1966).

The present study clearly indicates a close positive association
between absence petit mal and awakening grand mal (Table 24 and
Figure 5). A negative association is also apparent with psychomotor and cortical epilepsy, grand mal during sleep, and with
diffuse and occasional grand mal.

Myoclonic Petit Mal. Patients with myoclonic petit mal revealed
a common association with grand mal (64 - 100 %; JANZ and
CHRISTIAN, 1957; HORI, 1959; DALBY, 1969; AICARDI and CHEVRIE,
1970). The grand mal was mainly of the awakening type (84 %:
JANZ and CHRISTIAN, 1957) and not cortical (HORI, 1959; DALBY,
1969), whereas the grand mal in patients with myoclonus epilepsy
usually occurred during sleep (JANZ, 1969).

The results of the authors' study indicate a positive association
of myoclonic petit mal with awakening grand mal, and a negative
association with four types of seizure: psychomotor epilepsy,
grand mal during sleep, and diffuse and occasional grand mal.

Awakening Grand Mal. Grand Mal during Sleep, and Diffuse Grand
Mal. A physiologic relationship between awakening grand mal and
absence petit mal has generally been assumed (JANZ, 1953; BEYER
and JOVANOVIC, 1966). According to CHRISTIAN (1961), patients
with awakening grand mal were frequently found to also have
associated petit mal triad (85 %). In comparison with the authors'

calculations, their findings were significantly higher than in
our patients with grand mal during sleep (16 %). The latter
group was more closely associated with psychomotor epilepsy
than was the former (15 % vs. 84 %).

No difference of association patterns were evident among the
three types of grand mal (FURUICHI, 1969).

Psychomotor Epilepsy. Patients with psychomotor epilepsy had
frequently associated grand mal during sleep (JANZ, 1969); however, according to our calculations, the difference of association
patterns with the three types of grand mal was not statistically
significant (awakening grand mal 15 %, S-GM 26 %, D-GM 24 %).
CHRISTIAN (1968) suggested the possibility that psychomotor
epilepsy might be subordinate to grand mal during sleep. However,
it has been stated that only 5 % of 666 patients with psychomotor
epilepsy had S-GM (Editorial, 1971). MEYER-MICKELEIT (1953) reported a frequency of 15 %.

The authors' analysis disclosed a negative association with four
types of seizure: Lennox syndrome, myoclonic and absence petit
mal, and awakening grand mal. No correlation was found with grand
mal during sleep, or with occasional or diffuse grand mal.

Cortical Epilepsy. Forty-seven percent of all patients with cortical epilepsy had grand mal (KRUSE, 1964). Although association
with any type of seizure was found to be possible in the authors'
study, there was a negative association with five types of seizure: absence and myoclonic peti mal, awakening grand mal, grand
mal during sleep, and diffuse grand mal.

13. Characteristic Finding in Each Type of Seizure

Comparisons were made between patients with certain types of
seizure and those with other types of seizure. All findings
characteristic for each type of seizure for the total number of
patients are summarized in Table 25. The χ^2 value has been described previously in this chapter. Male as well as female patients sometimes showed other inverse results; these factors
are reported in detail in the appropriate chapters.

13.1. Awakening Grand Mal

Compared with those with other types of seizure, patients with
A-GM showed an increased frequency of seizures between 15 and
24 years of age (41 %); 85 % were 10 - 39 years of age. The frequency of onset of seizure between 6 and 22 years of age was
increased (78 %). There was an increased frequency in patients
with typical sp-w-c (12 %), in atypical sp-w-c (20 %), in 2-2.5/s
sp-w-c (4.8 %), in 3.5-5/s sp-w-c (9.5 %), in multiple sp-w-c
(16 %), and in those with total sp-w-c (33 %). Of the total number of patients, 71 % had paroxysmal EEG patterns. The patients
with high voltage α-rhythm was higher in incidence (14 %) and

those with pathologic findings during hyperventilation were also
higher (42 %). Only 6.8 % of the patients showed focal sign in
EEG. A higher frequency of patients with familial predisposition
to epilepsy (11 %) was observed; on the other hand, the frequency
of patients with exogenous factors was found to be lower (7.5 %)
than in patients with other types of seizure.

In the association analysis, A-GM was found to have a positive
correlation with both absence PM and myoclonic PM, and a negative
correlation with four types: S-GM, D-GM, and psychomotor and
cortical epilepsy.

13.2. Grand Mal During Sleep

This type of seizure occurred significantly more frequently in
the aged, particularly in patients over 45 years of age (24 %);
60 % of the patients were male. The age at onset was 11 - 25 years
in 48 % of patients and the frequency in onset over 35 years was
23 %. There was only one patient with atypical sp-w-c (1.1 %),
none with typical sp-w-c or with multiple sp-w-c. Compared with
those with other types of seizures, patients with S-GM revealed
a decreased frequency of paroxysmal EEG patterns (46 %). The
incidence of patients with high voltage α-rhythm and β-EEG (10 %)
was lower. The frequency of patients with pathologic findings
during hyperventilation was lower; 17 % of patients showed focal
sign in EEG. A lower frequency of familial predisposition to
epilepsy (6.7 %) and of the presence of exogenous factors (6.7 %)
was found.

In the association analysis, S-GM indicated a negative correlation with five types of seizure: A-GM, Lennox syndrome, absence
and myoclonic petit mal, and cortical epilepsy. No type of seizure had a positive correlation with S-GM. The association between S-GM and psychomotor seizure was not as close as had been
assumed in previous studies.

13.3. Diffuse Grand Mal

Compared with those with other types of seizures, patients with
D-GM revealed an increased frequency in the age group over 35
years (38 %); 61 % were male. Frequency increased in patients
with the age of onset of 0 - 4 years (18 %). There was a decreased
frequency in patients with paroxysmal EEG patterns (52 %) and in
total sp-w-c (7.3 %). A decrease was observed in the incidence
of patients with high voltage α-rhythm and in those with pathologic findings during hyperventilation. Patients with a higher
frequency of focal sign were observed (20 %). A lower frequency
of patients with familial predisposition to epilepsy (7.3 %),
but a higher frequency of the presence of exogenous factors
(16 %), was found.

The association analysis indicated a negative correlation with
four types of seizure: A-GM, Lennox syndrome, myoclonic petit mal,
and cortical epilepsy. No positive association were found.

13.4. Occasional Grand Mal

No characteristic findings concerning the distribution of patients
by age, sex, onset, paroxysmal EEG abnormalities, and familial
predisposition to epilepsy were observed. Higher incidence were
found in patients with low voltage EEG (11 %) and in the presence
of exogenous factors (18 %) in patients with occasional grand
mal than in those with other types of seizures.

13.5. West Syndrome and Lennox Syndrome

In the authors' study, only 3 patients were clinically diagnosed
to have West syndrome and 5 patients diagnosed with Lennox syndrome. Because of the small number of patients, the authors were
unable to draw any definite conclusions. However, compared with
patients with other types of seizures, a higher incidence of patients with high voltage α-rhythm and a lower incidence of exogenous factors (40 %) were found in patients with Lennox syndrome.
The frequency of patients with atypical sp-w-c was higher (60 %),
and all patients had paroxysmal activity.

In the association analysis, a negative association was found between Lennox syndrome and both absence PM and psychomotor epilepsy. There were no positive associations.

13.6. Absence Petit Mal

Compared with patients with other types of seizures, patients
with absence PM showed an increased frequency in the 5 - 24-year-
old age group (63 %). The distribution of patients by age at
onset of seizure was higher at 5 - 17 years (83 %). EEG examinations demonstrated an increased frequency in patients with typical
sp-w-c (19 %), in atypical sp-w-c (19 %), in 3.5-5/s sp-w-c (11 %),
in multiple sp-w-c (19 %), and in patients with total sp-w-c
(37 %). Paroxysmal EEG activity occurred in 73 % of our patients.
A higher incidence of patients with high voltage α-rhythm (13 %),
and of β-EEG (21 %), but no patient with low voltage EEG and a
lower frequency of patients with focal sign (5.7 %) were found.
There was an increased frequency of patients with pathologic
findings during hyperventilation (51 %). The frequency of patients
with familial predisposition to epilepsy was higher in frequency
(21 %), while the frequency of those with exogenous factors was
lower (2.9 %).

In the association analysis, a positive association was found between absence PM and A-GM; however, there was a negative association between absence PM and S-GM, and with psychomotor or cortical
epilepsy.

13.7. Myoclonic Petit Mal

All patients were 10 - 39 years of age. Compared with those with
other types of seizures patients with myoclonic PM had the in-

creased frequency of patients with age at onset of seizure in
the age group of 10 - 16 years (71 %); 82 % showed paroxysmal EEG
patterns. The frequency observed was increased in patients with
typical sp-w-c (17 %), in multiple sp-w-c (17 %), in atypical
sp-w-c (31 %), and in those with total sp-w-c (49 %). The incidence of patients with β-EEG was higher (40 %). A higher incidence of patients with high voltage α-rhythm (14 %), but a lower
incidence of patients with slow waves (23 %) as well as focal
sign (5.7 %) was found. The frequency of patients with familial
predisposition to epilepsy was slightly higher (11 %); however,
that of the presence of exogenous factors was lower (11 %).

In the association analysis, a positive association was found
between myoclonic PM and A-GM, but a negative association was
observed with three types of seizures: S-GM, D-GM, and psychomotor epilepsy.

13.8. Total Petit Mal

Compared with patients with other types of seizures, patients
with any type of petit mal demonstrated an increased frequency
in the group 5 - 29 years of age (72 %). A higher frequency of
female patients was found in total PM. The first seizure occurred
in 79 % of patients in the age range of 5 - 17 years. The EEG examination of patients with this type of seizure indicated an increased frequency in paroxysmal activity (77 %), in typical sp-w-c
(18 %), in atypical sp-w-c (27 %), in 2-2.5/s sp-w-c (6.6 %), in
3.5-5/s sp-w-c (12 %), in multiple sp-w-c (20 %), and in those
with total sp-w-c (45 %). Concerning individual EEG patterns,
there was an increased incidence in patients with β-EEG (26 %),
and in pathologic findings during hyperventilation (52 %) but a
decrease in the occurrence of focal sign (7.5 %). A high incidence of patients with high voltage α-rhythm (13 %) was observed,
but there was no patient with low voltage EEG. The frequency of
patients with familial predisposition to epilepsy was higher
(18 %); on the other hand, the incidence of exogenous factors
was lower (6.6 %).

13.9. Psychomotor Epilepsy

The ages of patients with psychomotor epilepsy varied widely.
Compared with patients with other types of seizures, patients
with psychomotor epilepsy revealed a higher frequency at 5 - 14
years of age (13 %) and over 50 years (15 %). The age at onset
of seizure was higher in frequency in patients between 0 - 15
years (21 %) and 20 - 29 years (25 %). The frequency of EEG abnormality was found to be lower in patients with typical sp-w-c
(1.7 %), in atypical sp-w-c (5.9 %), in total sp-w-c (7.6 %),
in 3.5-5/s sp-w-c (0.8 %), and in those with multiple sp-w-c
(1.7 %). A most remarkable finding was the increase in patients
with temporal discharge (9.2 %). Focal sign in EEG was also increased (30 %). Patients with predisposition to epilepsy was
lower in frequency (6.7 %).

In the association analysis, a negative association only was observed between psychomotor epilepsy and A-GM, absence PM, myoclonic PM, Lennox syndrome, and with cortical epilepsy.

13.10. Cortical Epilepsy

Patients with cortical epilepsy showed less marked findings. There was only an increase in the incidence of exogenous factors (32.5 %); 73 % was males.

In the association analysis, the authors observed only a negative association with five types of seizure: A-GM, S-GM, D-GM, absence PM, and psychomotor epilepsy.

14. Comparison of Characteristic Findings Observed in Each Type of Seizure

The characteristic findings found with each type of seizure are discussed in the following section.

14.1. Awakening Grand Mal, Absence Petit Mal, and Myoclonic Petit Mal

Patients with A-GM, absence PM, and with myoclonic PM revealed some similar characteristic findings, such as: (1) the onset of seizure was mainly at puberty or prepuberty; (2) nearly all of our patients revealed paroxysmal EEG patterns, especially typical and atypical sp-w-c; (3) the basic EEG rhythm showed a high incidence of (a) high voltage α-rhythm, (b) β-EEG, (c) pathologic findings during hyperventilation, and a low incidence of focal sign; (4) familial predisposition to epilepsy was higher in incidence, and that of the presence of exogenous factors was inversely lower; and (5) in the association analysis, patients with these types of seizures showed many similarities as indicated above.

In previous studies, only a few authors have stated the difference in EEG between patients with grand mal and those with absence petit mal as follows: the patients with absence petit mal showed more typical sp-w-c, the amplitude of spikes was more stable, the amplitude of slow waves was greater, and the duration of sp-w-c was longer than in patients with grand mal.

14.2. Comparison Between Patients with Pure Awakening Grand Mal, and Associated Absence or Myoclonic Petit Mal (Table 26)

Since patients with awakening grand mal were associated positively with either absence petit mal (45/147, 31 %) or myoclonic petit mal (24/147, 16 %), the authors compared three patient groups: pure A-GM, absence PM, and with myoclonic PM.

Compared with those with pure type of A-GM, patients with absence petit mal revealed an increased frequency of age at onset of seizure between O and 9 years (60 % vs. 9.4 %, P < 0.001) and 3/s sp-w-c (19 % vs. 3.8 %, P < 0.05). Compared with those with pure type of A-GM, patients with myoclonic petit mal indicated an increased frequency of age at onset of seizure between O and 9 years (30 % vs. 9.4 %, P < 0.05), and β-EEG (42 % vs. 17 %, P < 0.01).

14.3. Absence Petit Mal and Myoclonic Petit Mal

Patients with absence petit mal and those with myoclonic petit mal had the following marked similar findings: (1) the distribution of patients by age was found mainly in the 5 - 29 year age group and many female patients experienced onset of seizure in puberty or prepuberty; (2) EEG examination indicated an increased frequency of paroxysmal EEG abnormalities, including typical as well as atypical sp-w-c; (3) a high incidence of β-EEG existed in the basic EEG rhythm, as well as pathologic findings during hyperventilation, and a low frequency of focal sign; and (4) a high frequency of familial predisposition to epilepsy and conversely a low frequency of the presence of exogenous factors.

Some of these findings were more marked in patients with absence PM. The age at onset of seizures in myoclonic PM was shifted toward adulthood. The only differences observed were a higher frequency of the age at onset of seizure between O and 9 years in patients with absence petit mal compared to those with myoclonic petit mal (60 % vs. 9 %, P < 0.001), and an increase of β-EEG in patients with myoclonic petit mal compared with those with absence PM (40% vs. 21 %, P < 0.05).

14.4. Awakening Grand Mal and Grand Mal During Sleep (Table 27)

When patients with A-GM and those with S-GM were compared, the following differences became apparent: (1) Compared with patients with S-GM, patients with A-GM were younger, the age at onset under 19 years was increased (77 % vs. 56 %, P < 0.001), but more older patients were found in the S-GM group; (2) in the A-GM group, the age at onset of seizures was increased between 6 and 22 years, but this was high over 35 years of age in S-GM group; (3) the frequency of paroxysmal EEG abnormalities (71 % vs. 46 %, P < 0.001) and sp-w-c (33 % vs. 1.1 %, P < 0.001) was higher in patients with A-GM than in those with S-GM. There were no patients with typical sp-w-c and only one patient with atypical sp-w-c in the S-GM group; (4) in the A-GM group, the incidence of high voltage α-rhythm (14 % vs. 4.5 %, P < 0.05), β-EEG (20 % vs. 10 %, P < 0.05), pathologic findings during hyperventilation (42 % vs. 11 %, P < 0.001), and familial predisposition to epilepsy was higher; the incidence of focal sign (6.8 % vs. 17 %, P < 0.05) was lower in the A-GM group than in those with S-GM; (5) the only similar finding with both types of GM was the low frequency of the presence of exogenous factors.

Association analysis indicated a negative association between patients with A-GM and those with S-GM. As shown above, in spite of a similar phenotype of grand mal both in A-GM and S-GM, these syndromes are quite heterogenous in many aspects. The difference in EEG and sleep-awake-rhythm (CHRISTIAN, 1961), the age at onset of seizure (JANZ, 1969), and psychologic findings (LEDER, 1969) between patients with A-GM and those with S-GM have been reported in previous studies.

14.5. Awakening Grand Mal and Diffuse Grand Mal

A similar correlation between the A-GM and D-GM groups was observed as between the A-GM and S-GM groups. For example, patients with diffuse grand mal decreased in frequency with respect to age at onset of 0 - 19 years (60 % vs. 77 %, P < 0.01), paroxysmal EEG abnormalities (52 % vs. 71 %, P < 0.01), sp-w-c (7.3 % vs. 33 %, P < 0.001) and pathologic changes during hyperventilation (24 % vs. 42 %, P < 0.01), whereas only the frequency of focal sign in EEG was higher (20 % vs. 6.8 %, P < 0.01). Association analysis also revealed similar findings to those observed between patients with A-GM and those with S-GM.

14.6. Awakening Grand Mal and Occasional Grand Mal

Compared with patients with A-GM, patients with occasional grand mal were lower in frequency with respect to age at onset of 0 - 19 years (53 % vs. 77 %, P < 0.001), in sp-w-c (15 % vs. 33 %, P < 0.01), and in paroxysmal EEG abnormality (53 % vs. 71 %, P < 0.001). On the other hand, an increased frequency was found in the presence of exogenous factors (18 % vs. 7.5 %, P < 0.05).

14.7. Grand Mal During Sleep and Diffuse Grand Mal

The following similar interesting findings were observed in patients with S-GM and in those with D-GM. Compared with patients with other types of seizures, (1) patients with S-GM or D-GM were frequently aged patients; (2) there was a lower frequency of paroxysmal EEG patterns, especially sp-w-c; (3) in the basic EEG rhythm, there was a lower incidence of high voltage α-rhythm and β-EEG; pathologic findings during hyperventilation and family predisposition to epilepsy were observed in low frequency in both groups; (4) a difference in frequencies existed only in (a) age at onset of seizure, (b) presence of exogenous factors (6.7 % vs. 16 %), and (c) pathologic changes during hyperventilation (11 % vs. 24 %, P < 0.05).

In the association analysis, the authors failed to find any positive association between patients with S-GM and those with D-GM; however, their association patterns to other types of seizure were quite similar, as shown in Table 24 and Figure 5.

14.8. Grand Mal During Sleep and Occasional Gand Mal

Similar distribution by different categories was observed in both groups. However, in patients with occasional grand mal the frequency of the presence of exogenous factors (18 % vs. 6.7 %, $P < 0.05$), sp-w-c (15 % vs. 1.1 %, $P < 0.01$), and pathologic changes during hyperventilation (29 % vs. 11 %, $P < 0.01$) were higher than in those with S-GM.

14.9. Diffuse Grand Mal and Occasional Grand Mal

No marked differences were observed in the distribution between the two groups.

14.10. Comparison Among Patients with Three Types of Seizure: Pure Grand Mal of Awakening, During Sleep, and Diffuse Types (Table 28)

Patients with three types of pure grand mal showed a distribution by EEG, familial predisposition to epilepsy, and exogenous factors similar to that found in the total number of types. The frequency of paroxysmal EEG abnormality in patients with awakening grand mal was higher compared to that in patients with grand mal during sleep (68 % vs. 36 %, $P < 0.01$) and also compared to that in patients with diffuse grand mal (68 % vs. 42 %, $P < 0.05$). Pathologic changes during hyperventilation in patients with diffuse grand mal were lower compared to those in patients with awakening grand mal (13 % vs. 36 %, $P < 0.05$) and also in patients with grand mal during sleep (13 % vs. 32 %, $P < 0.05$).

14.11. West Syndrome and Lennox Syndrome

Since both groups contained a relatively small number of patients, no definite conclusions can be reported.

STÖGMANN and LORENZONI (1970) studied 54 patients with Blitz-Nick-Salaamkrämpfe (West syndrome), and divided them into two groups: (1) 47 patients with cerebral damage, and (2) 7 patients without it. In the first group of patients, Blitz- and Salaamkrämpfe were more common as a type of seizure, onset of disease was earlier and a higher incidence of neuropsychiatric symptoms and combinations with grand mal were found. Seventy percent showed hypsarrhythmia and there was a low frequency of family predisposition to epilepsy. The second group of patients revealed

different features: the <u>Nick-Krampf</u> type of seizure was more
common; onset of seizures was later; no neuropsychiatric symptoms
were evident; a higher frequency of familial predisposition to
epilepsy was present, the disease was most often combined with
Lennox syndrome, and generalized paroxysmal EEG abnormalities
were demonstrated.

14.12. Comparison Between Patients With Combined Petit Mal and Those With Uncombined Pure Petit Mal

One hundred and six patients with petit mal were divided into
two groups: 90 combined with other types of seizures and 16 uncombined pure petit mal.

Both groups demonstrated a very similar distribution by age at
onset of seizures, paroxysmal EEG abnormalities, basic EEG rhythm,
familial predisposition to epilepsy, and exogenous factors, as
shown in Table 29. A higher incidence of β-EEG and slow waves in
the pure petit mal group was evident. A statistically significant
difference was found only in patients with 3/s sp-w-c (19 % vs.
0 %, P(Fisher) = 0.032).

14.13. Psychomotor Epilepsy and Awakening Grand Mal

There were no similar findings between patients with A-GM and
those with psychomotor epilepsy. A marked dissimilarity was found
in distribution by age, onset, EEG abnormalities, pathologic
findings during hyperventilation, and focal sign (30 % vs. 6.8 %,
see Table 25, P < 0.001).

In the association analysis, patients with psychomotor epilepsy
showed a negative association with those with A-GM, absence PM,
myoclonic PM, Lennox syndrome, and with cortical epilepsy.

14.14. Psychomotor Epilepsy, S-GM, and D-GM

Similar interesting findings were observed in patients with
psychomotor epilepsy, S-GM, and with D-GM as follows: (1) a
higher frequency of aged patients and focal sign in EEG; and
(2) a lower frequency of typical as well as atypical sp-w-c,
familial predisposition to epilepsy, and exogenous factors than
in those with other types of seizures. No dissimilar findings
were observed.

In the association analysis, no positive association could be
found, although the association patterns were very similar.

14.15. Comparison Between Patients With Combined, Uncombined Psychomotor Epilepsy, Uncombined Grand Mal During Sleep, and With Pure Diffuse Grand Mal

Patients with psychomotor epilepsy were divided into two groups, combined and uncombined. There was no marked difference between the two groups with respect to sex, age at onset of seizure, paroxysmal EEG abnormalities, basic EEG rhythm, familial pre-disposition to epilepsy, and the presence of exogenous factors, as shown in Table 30. A difference existed only in the incidence of β-EEG (37.5 % vs. 13.7 %, $P < 0.01$).

Patients with uncombined psychomotor epilepsy were compared with those with uncombined grand mal during sleep and those with pure diffuse grand mal. Patients with uncombined psychomotor epilepsy showed a higher frequency of age at onset between 0 and 9 years, pathologic changes during hyperventilation, an increase of par-oxysmal EEG abnormalities (71 % vs. 36 %, $P < 0.05$, compared with patients with pure S-GM; 71 % vs. 42 %, $P < 0.05$, compared with those with pure diffuse GM) and β-EEG (38 % vs. 2.6 %, $P < 0.001$, compared with those with pure S-GM). Pathologic changes during hyperventilation were higher in frequency in pa-tients with uncombined D-GM than in those with uncombined S-GM (33 % vs. 13 %, $P < 0.05$).

14.16. Psychomotor Epilepsy, Absence Petit Mal, and Myoclonic Petit Mal

Patients with absence PM and those with myoclonic PM revealed very similar findings to those with A-GM, almost the same as the correlation between patients with psychomotor epilepsy and those with A-GM indicated.

14.17. Cortical Epilepsy

As mentioned above, patients with cortical epilepsy showed less marked findings. Compared with patients with other types of sei-zures, patients with cortical epilepsy exhibit only an increased frequency of focal sign in EEG (33 %) and the presence of exo-genous factors (33 %).

According to the results of association analysis, there is no close correlation between patients with cortical epilepsy and any other types of seizure.

15. Discussion and Summary

Previous authors indicated the presence of a close correlation between certain types of seizures and certain corresponding par-oxysmal EEG abnormalities such as West syndrome and hypsarrhythmia

(GIBBS and GIBBS, 1952), Lennox syndrome and slow sp-w-c
(KRUSE, 1968), absence or pure petit mal and 3/s sp-w-c (JASPER
and KERSCHMAN, 1941), pyknoleptic petit mal and 3/s sp-w-c
(BAMBERGER and MATTHES, 1959), myoclonic epilepsy or myoclonic
(impulsive) petit mal and multiple sp-w-c (JASPER and KERSCHMAN,
1941; PENFIELD, 1954; JANZ and CHRISTIAN, 1957), awakening grand
mal and 3-4/s sp-w-c or paroxysmal dysrhythmia (GÄNSHIRT and
VETTER, 1961), grand mal during sleep and a low incidence of
specific as well as paroxysmal abnormalities, but a markedly
high rate of sleep provocation (CHRISTIAN, 1961), psychomotor
epilepsy and focal temporal discharge (GLASER and GOLUB, 1955),
and cortical or focal epilepsy and focal discharge (SILVERMAN,
1954).

All of these studies were done in patients with a specific type
of seizure and those with a special type of EEG abnormality. The
present authors have taken a large randomly selected group of
epileptic patients to analyze a correlation between clinical
type of seizure and specific EEG abnormality. The results observed in the present study have confirmed the findings of previous studies mentioned above. By coefficient contingency analysis, a positive correlation (relative coefficient of contingency
$c_r > +0.5$) was found between: awakening GM and 3/s sp-w-c, as
well as multiple sp-w-c; absence and 3/s sp-w-c; myoclonic petit
mal and total paroxysmal abnormalities; Lennox syndrome and atypical sp-w-c, as well as sharp wave; and psychomotor epilepsy and
temporal discharge. A negative correlation (relative coefficient
of contingency $c_r < -0.5$) was observed between: GM during sleep
and 3/s, atypical, slow, 3.5-5/s, as well as multiple sp-w-c;
diffuse GM and atypical, slow, and 3.5-5/s sp-w-c; myoclonic
petit mal and temporal discharge; psychomotor epilepsy and 3/s,
3.5-5/s, and multiple sp-w-c; cortical epilepsy and total sp-w-c;
and Lennox syndrome and temporal discharge.

The results observed in the authors' study support those of previous reports. All possible correlations were first made by the
authors using a statistical analysis in a large randomly selected
group of epileptic patients.

An increased frequency of focal EEG abnormality was observed in
patients with some types of seizures, such as psychomotor epilepsy
as reported by NIEDERMEYER (1957), cortical epilepsy as found by
KRUSE (1964), and West syndrome (STÖGMANN and LORENZONI, 1970).
On the other hand, a lower frequency was found in patients with
absence or pyknoleptic petit mal (JANZ, 1955; BAMBERGER and
MATTHES, 1959), myoclonic petit mal (JANZ and CHRISTIAN, 1957),
and awakening GM (CHRISTIAN, 1961; KRISCHEK, 1962). The increase
of focal abnormality in patients with different age groups may
be heterogenous in etiology.

Concerning the frequency of familial predisposition in patients
with different types of seizures, a large variety has been reported previously. In general, a higher frequency was found in
patients with absence or pure petit mal than in others, as found
in the present study. GIBBS and GIBBS (1952) also found that
patients with focal seizure revealed a lower frequency of familial
predisposition.

A close correlation between type of seizure and exogenous factors
was observed. That is, a lower frequency of exogenous factors
was confirmed in patients with A-GM, absence PM, and myoclonic
PM, whereas the frequency increased in patients with focal seizure, Lennox syndrome, diffuse GM, as well as occasional GM.
These findings correspond to those observed by previous authors
as described in Chapter III.11.

The occurrence of more than one type of clinical seizure seems
to be much higher than was assumed previously. The figure in the
present study is 51 %.

Simultaneous or later occurrence of certain types of seizures
in the same individuals was noted by previous authors:

1. Absence and grand mal: a high frequency (38 - 69 %) of patients
with pure petit mal as well as absence had, simultaneously or
later, grand mal (SACHS and HAUSMAN, 1926; BRIDGE, 1949; GASTAUT,
1954; CLARK and KNOTT, 1955; CALDERON and PAAL, 1957; LENNOX and
LENNOX, 1960; HOLOWACH et al., 1962; LIVINGSTON et al., 1965;
GIBBERD, 1966; DALBY, 1969; PAZZAGLIA et al., 1971; 64 % in the
present study).

2. Absence or pyknoleptic petit mal and awakening grand mal:
JANZ (1955) reported that 53 % of patients with pyknoleptic PM
were affected with GM, and 88 % of patients with GM was of the
awakening type (64 % and 90 %, respectively, in the present
study).

3. Myoclonic petit mal and awakening grand mal: of 47 patients
with impulsive petit mal 42 had A-GM (JANZ and CHRISTIAN, 1957).
This figure was 73 % in the present study. DALBY (1969) found
that 86 % of his patients with myoclonic PM had GM, but none
showed focal seizure.

4. Lennox syndrome and absence or grand mal: Many patients with
Lennox syndrome had absence or GM (LANCE, 1969; BUENO et al.,
1970; SCHNEIDER et al., 1970).

5. West syndrome and GM during sleep: JANZ and MATTHES (1955).

6. Psychomotor epilepsy and GM during sleep: CHRISTIAN (1968).
In the present study, 26 % of the patients with psychomotor
epilepsy had GM during sleep.

7. Grand mal during sleep and focal seizure: KRUSE (1964). In
the present study only 4 % of patients with S-GM had cortical
seizures.

The results outlined in the studies noted above have been confirmed by the authors. On the basis of the results mentioned
above and others and also the present multidimensional analysis,
it may be concluded that there exist at least five neurophysi-
ologic subgroups in epilepsies. They are (1) awakening grand
mal, myoclonic petit mal, and absence or pyknoleptic petit mal,
(2) grand mal during sleep, (3) diffuse grand mal, (4) psychomotor epilepsy, and (5) cortical or focal epilepsy. Although
some similarities exist among them with respect to phenotypical
expressions, they are quite different in etiology, age at onset
of seizure, paroxysmal EEG abnormalities, basic EEG rhythm, etc.

Significant findings in patients with each type of seizure were
reported in Chapter III.13. Their characteristic features are
summarized in Table 25. Among 10 clinical types of seizure some
similarities and dissimilarities concerning different factors
were observed. After comparing those findings, they were sepa-
rated into 5 groups, as mentioned above, mainly on the basis of
age at onset, pathologic EEG findings, clinical association,
familial predisposition, and exogenous factors.

In previous studies, some patients with petit mal were found to
develop grand mal (GASTAUT, 1954). This correlation was analyzed
in 79 patients with petit mal and grand mal with regard to evolution of type of seizure and time of occurrence.

IV. Age at Onset of Seizure

1. General Outline

The distribution of male and female patients by age at onset of
seizure is shown in Table 3, and the cumulated sum of the per-
centages is illustrated in Figure 1.

The distribution of patients by age at onset of seizure according
to type of seizure is shown in Tables 11 and 12. Irrespective of
type of seizure, male patients (Figure 2a) showed an initial peak
at age 0-1 year, thereafter decreasing until age 4 years. Of
the total male patients, the highest incidence was found in the
age group 8-17 years (38 %). The peak age of onset was seen at
age 10 and 12 years, thereafter gradually decreasing.

In female patients (Figure 2c), an initial peak at infancy was
not observed. Incidence rapidly increased at age 4 years, reaching
an initial peak at age 6-7 years. A second peak occurred at age
12-13 years. The highest frequencies were seen at age 6-15
years (44 %), followed by a gradual decrease in incidence. At
age 38-39 years, however, the frequency of onset of seizures
was again markedly increased.

The distribution in the total number of patients can be seen in
Figure 2e. The initial peak was found and the highest frequencies
observed at ages 6-15 years (39 %). Thereafter incidence decreased with age.

Male and female patients were compared with respect to onset of
seizures: (1) the initial peak at age 0-1 year was found only
in male patients, (2) the highest frequencies were found earlier
in females than in males, (3) a bimodal distribution was found
only in females, (4) the distribution curve revealed a more rapid
rise to the peak and a more sharp downturn in female patients,
(5) the number of female patients at the peak was greater than
the number of male patients, and (6) a small projection at age
38-39 years was observed only in female patients.

The correlation between type of seizure and age at onset of seizure has been discussed in Chapter III. Only a few reports in
the literature are available to compare with the results of the
present study. TAEN et al. (1956) reported that age at onset of
seizure occurred with a frequency of 65 % between 10 and 25 years
of age in their group of epileptic patients, nearly all of whom
were adults. The validity of this figure obviously depends on
the group of patients under study, i.e., age distribution, type
of seizures, etc. Such figures are, therefore, quite different
when reported for adult epileptics and for child epileptics.

In previous studies the incidence of late onset epilepsy has
been reported as between 1.7 and 9.5 % by different authors
(1.7 % after age 50: LENNOX and LENNOX, 1960; 3.7 % after age
45: KUHLO and SCHWARZ, 1971; 4 % after age 50: WHITE et al.,
1953; 6.5 % after age 45: HYLLESTED and PAKKENBERG, 1963; 9.5 %
after age 40: MAYER and TRÜBESTEIN, 1968). In the present study,
the figures are 7.7 % after age 40, 4.7 % after age 45, 2.4 %
after age 50, and 1.1 % after 60 years of age.

2. Age at Onset of Seizure and Sex

Distribution by age at onset of seizure between 2 and 9 years
in female patients was higher than in male patients (30 % vs.
19 %, P < 0.01). This result might be correlated with the female
predominance, especially during childhood and preadolescence,
with absence petit mal. On the other hand, very early onset —
0 - 1 year of age — occurred predominantly in males (70 %). This
might be correlated with the male predominance in early childhood epilepsy, for example, in West and Lennox syndromes as
mentioned in Chapter II. Onset at an age of over 40 years was
found more often in male than in female patients (9.1 % vs. 5.8 %).
Among late-onset epileptics, male patients were also predominant
(72 % vs. 28 % according to NIEDERMEYER, 1958; 63 % vs. 37 %
according to KUHLO and SCHWARZ, 1971). These findings correspond
with those in the present study (69 % vs. 31 %).

The mean age at onset was 18.7 ± S.E. 0.05 for males, 17.0 ± 0.07
for females, and 18.3 ± 0.03 years for the total number of patients. The differences are not statistically significant.

3. Age at Onset of Seizure and Type of Seizure

The correlations between each type of seizure and the age at onset of disease were analyzed separately.

3.1. Male Patients

Correlations are shown in Table 11 and Figure 2b. The peak of
distribution by age at onset in patients with A-GM was found in

the 8 - 11-year-old group; incidence thereafter rapidly decreased.
Incidence was widely distributed over age 0 - 48 years, but principally between 6 and 23 years (63/84, 75 %). Four patients had
their first attack of A-GM between the age of 42 - 48 years. The
distribution in patients with S-GM ranged from 0 - 60 years. The
peak incidence was found at 14 - 15 years, 4 - 6 years later than
that found in patients with A-GM. The characteristic finding was,
that the incidence of S-GM was distributed well beyond 40 years
of age. In patients with D-GM, the first peak of incidence was
noted at age 0 - 1 year and a second peak at 12 - 13 years. A peak
in the incidence of O-GM also occurred at age 12 - 13 years. In
general, the distribution of age at onset in patients with S-GM,
D-GM, and O-GM varied widely and after a peak was reached, the
rate of incidence gradually decreased with age.

The distribution of patients with absence PM was very limited,
with a peak found in the age group of 4 - 11 years (maximum 8 - 11
years). Only 2 patients were more than 18 years of age. The curve
was similar to that in patients with A-GM and the peak occurred
at the same age. The distribution of patients with myoclonic PM
was found to be similar to that observed in patients with absence
PM, but the myoclonic PM group shifted slightly toward adulthood.

Patients with psychomotor epilepsy showed a diffuse distribution
from 0 - 60 years, with the most frequent distribution being in
the age group 12 - 23 years. The highest peak was observed in the
0 - 1 year age group, a finding characteristic to that found in
patients with D-GM. This might be correlated with the findings
in the association analysis between type of seizure in the same
individual noted in Chapter III. A combination of psychomotor
epilepsy and D-GM might be found in these cases.

3.2. Female Patients

The correlations are shown in Table 12 and Figure 2d. Patients
with A-GM ranged from 0 - 31 years, with the peak observed in
the 12 - 15 year group. The distribution in the total patients
with S-GM, D-GM, and O-GM ranged widely from 0 - 60 years. A peak
was found at 6 - 7 years, but it was not as high as that found in
patients with A-GM. After peaking, the rate of incidence decreased
very gradually. The smallest peak was observed at 38 - 39 years.
The peak of distribution of absence PM was seen in 6 - 7 year
group, with 66 % of patients developing absence PM between the
4 - 9 years. After this age, incidence decreased sharply. Four
patients had their first seizures after 20 years of age. The
peak of distribution of myoclonic PM was observed at age 14 - 15
years, corresponding to the peak found in patients with A-GM.

The distribution of patients with psychomotor and cortical epilepsy was widely observed. Some similarity in this distribution
was noted between patients with S-GM and those with psychomotor
epilepsy.

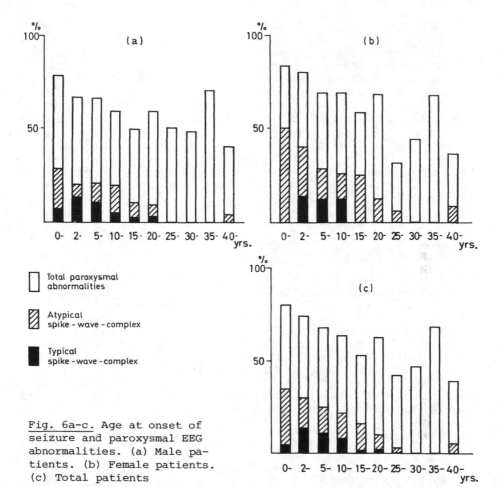

Fig. 6a-c. Age at onset of seizure and paroxysmal EEG abnormalities. (a) Male patients. (b) Female patients. (c) Total patients

3.3. Total Patients

The distribution of patients by age at onset of seizure in each type of seizure for the total number of patients was similar to that found in male and female patients as shown in Figure 2f. This correlation is further analyzed in Chapter IV.9.

3.4. Comparison Between Distribution by Age at Onset of Seizure in Male and Female Patients

In general, similar distribution by age at onset of seizure was seen in all types of seizures in both male and female patients.

4. Age at Onset of Seizure and Paroxysmal EEG Abnormalities

The correlation between age at onset of seizure and paroxysmal EEG patterns is shown in Table 31 and Figure 6a-c.

4.1. Male Patients

The frequency of paroxysmal EEG patterns was found to be highest
(79 %) in patients with onset at age 0 - 1 year; it decreased
gradually with age, declining to 40 % in the 40+ year age group.
Compared with patients with other age at onset, the frequency
of paroxysmal EEG patterns was higher in those with age at onset
between 0 and 9 years (69 % or 46 of 67, P < 0.05). After age
40 years, only one patient showed irregular sp-w-c. All but one
patient who had total sp-w-c had their first seizures before 24
years of age. The frequency of atypical sp-w-c was increased in
the group where age at onset occurred before 14 years (13 % or
16 of 125, P < 0.05) than in those with age at onset after 15
years (4 % or 6 of 151 patients).

4.2. Female Patients

The highest frequency of paroxysmal EEG patterns was found in
patients with age at onset between 0 and 1 year (83 %); it decreased with age and reached a minimum at age 25 - 29 years (31 %),
again showing a small peak between 35 and 39 years (67 %). The
frequency of paroxysmal EEG abnormality was higher in the group
with age at onset of 0 - 9 years (73 % or 46 of 63, P < 0.05) and
0 - 14 years (71 % or 75 of 105, P < 0.01) than in those with
other age at onset of seizures. Only one patient with sp-w-c was
over 30 at onset. The frequency of total sp-w-c was higher in
the group with age at onset of 0 - 14 years (30 % or 32 of 105,
P < 0.01) than in those with other age at onset of seizures.

4.3. Total Patients

The frequency of paroxysmal EEG patterns was higher in patients
with onset at 0 - 9 years (71 % or 92 of 130 patients, P < 0.01),
and 0 - 14 years (67 % or 155 of 230 patients, P < 0.001), while
it was lower when onset occurred at 40+ years (39 %, P < 0.01)
compared with those with other age at onset. The frequency of
sp-w-c in those where onset occurred during 0 - 14 years (25 %
or 58 of 230 patients, P < 0.001) was increased.

In previous studies, the incidence of EEG abnormality has been
observed to decrease linearly with age of onset from 0 - 9 until
40+ years (AJMONE MARSAN and ZIVIN, 1970). This tendency has
also been observed in epileptic children (ARIMA, 1959). Epileptic
children with a very early onset at age of 0 - 1 year frequently
showed hypsarrhythmia (29 %), 2/s sp-w-c (13 %), and focal spikes
or sp-w-c (12 %) (CAVAZZUTI et al., 1969). Late-onset epileptics
usually revealed diffuse or focal abnormalities (FISCHER, 1959;
HYLLESTED and PAKKENBERG, 1963; TAKAHASHI et al., 1965; OTOMO
and TSUBAKI, 1966; MAYER and TRÜBESTEIN, 1968; KUHLO and SCHWARZ,
1971). A bilateral generalized seizure potential was seldom found.

With respect to focal abnormality, there were some effects of
age. According to GABOR and AJMONE MARSAN (1969) patients with

bilateral focal EEG abnormality had a younger age at onset (average 9.7 years) than those with unilateral focus (14.5 years). This might be correlated with the finding that younger patients are more apt to have bilateral involvement and are more prone to hereditary influences as already described. This correlation is analyzed in Chapter IV.9.

4.4. Comparison Between Correlations Found in Male and Female Patients

As indicated in Table 31 and Figure 6, the distribution by frequencies of paroxysmal EEG patterns in male and in female patients were generally similar. A higher frequency of atypical sp-w-c was observed in female than in male patients (15.8 % vs. 8.0 %, P < 0.01). Other differences included the observation that the incidence curve in female patients was concave and the minimum of paroxysmal EEG abnormality was found in those patients with age at onset between 25 and 29 years.

5. Age at Onset of Seizure and Basic EEG Rhythm

5.1. α-EEG

The correlation between the age at onset of seizure and α-EEG is shown in Table 32.

5.1.1. Male Patients

The incidence of normal α-EEG was lower in those with age at onset of seizure between 5 and 14 years; thereafter, it increased with age in an inverse proportion to the incidence of slow waves. High voltage α-activity showed a higher incidence in the group with age of onset between 5 and 14 years; thereafter it decreased with age.

5.1.2. Female Patients

A similar distribution of the incidence of α-EEG to that found in male patients was observed, as shown in Table 32. In female patients the incidence of high-voltage α-EEG was higher (15 % vs. 6.9 %, P < 0.01) and normal α-EEG was lower (72 % vs. 84 %, P < 0.01) than in male patients.

5.1.3. Total Number of Patients

The incidence of normal α-EEG was lower in those with age of onset at 0 - 14 years (71 %, P < 0.05); the incidence of high-

voltage α-EEG was higher. However, the differences were not statistically significant.

5.2. β-EEG

The correlation between age at onset of seizure and β-EEG is
shown in Table 33.

5.2.1. Male Patients

Patients with β-EEG were rather diffusely distributed regardless
of age at onset of seizure between 0 and 40+ years; a somewhat
lower incidence was found in those with age at onset between 0
and 4 years (2 of 29 patients), but a higher incidence when age
of onset was between 5 and 9 years (24 %).

5.2.2. Female Patients

Distribution of patients by age at onset of seizure was more
limited than in male patients. More than 25 % of the patients
with their first seizure in the 5 - 29 year age groups showed
β-EEG. This was higher in incidence (28 % or 39 of 140 patients,
P < 0.01).

5.2.3. Total Number of Patients

Eighty-one patients showed β-EEG; the distribution was highest
in the group with age at onset of seizure of 5 - 19 years (22 %
or 53 of 243 patients, P < 0.01).

5.2.4. Comparison Between Findings in the Two Sexes

The incidence of β-EEG was higher in female than in male patients
(23 % vs. 14 %, P < 0.05). Distribution by age of onset of seizure was narrow in females, whereas in males it was more diffuse
with the highest incidence seen in those with earlier age of
onset of disease.

5.3. Slow Waves

The correlation between age at onset of seizure and incidence
of slow waves is shown in Table 34 and Figure 7. Patients with
θ-wave dominant EEG as well as θ-δ-wave dominant EEG are listed
under θ-δ-waves.

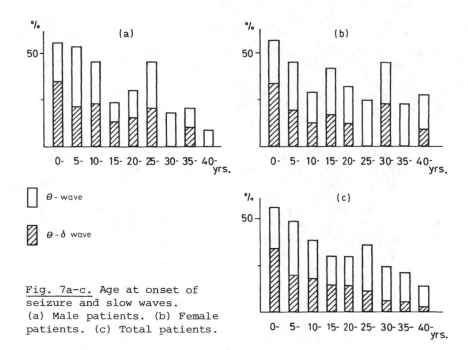

Fig. 7a-c. Age at onset of
seizure and slow waves.
(a) Male patients. (b) Female
patients. (c) Total patients.

5.3.1. Male Patients

The incidence of slow waves was highest in males between 0 and
4 years old at onset of disease; it decreased gradually thereafter. The incidence was higher in patients with age at onset
of seizure between 0 - 14 years (θ 25 %, θ + δ 50 %, P < 0.001)
and it decreased in patients over 30 years of age (θ 12 %, θ + δ
14 %, P < 0.001). The incidence of very slow (θ, δ) waves decreased in patients over 30 years of age.

5.3.2. Female Patients

There was an increased incidence of slow waves in female patients
with age at onset of seizure of 0 - 9 years (θ 25 %, θ + δ 49 %,
P < 0.05).

5.3.3. Total Number of Patients

Of the total patients with slow waves, the incidence was higher
with age at onset of 0 - 14 years (θ + δ 46 %, P < 0.001), particularly in the 0 - 9 year age group (θ + δ 52 %, P < 0.001).
This decreased after 30 years of age (θ + δ 20 %, P < 0.01),
mainly due to the decrease of θ - δ waves (4.6 %, P < 0.01).

5.3.4. Comparison Between Findings in Male and in Female Patients

In male patients, the incidence of slow waves tended to decrease with age, a distinction not clearly observed in female patients.

5.4. Low Voltage EEG

The correlation between age at onset of seizure and low voltage EEG is analyzed. Of the total number of patients observed, low voltage EEG were found mainly in patients with onset at 20 - 39 years of age (10 of 13 patients, P < 0.001), and also commonly female patients with onset in this age range (P(Fisher) = 0.0044). No patient with onset of 40+ years of age was found with low voltage EEG, and only 3 patients with onset at 9, 11, and 12 years of age were detected with this finding.

5.5. Pathologic Findings During Hyperventilation

The correlation between age at onset of seizure and pathologic EEG findings during hyperventilation was analyzed.

5.5.1. Male Patients

The frequency of pathologic findings during hyperventilation was higher in patients with onset at 0 - 9 years (45 % or 30 of 67 patients, P < 0.001) and in those with 0 - 14 years (38 % or 48 of 125 patients, P < 0.01), and decreased when age of onset was over 25 years (16 % or 12 of 77 patients, P < 0.01) than in those in other age groups at onset of disease.

5.5.2. Female Patients

There was an increased frequency in patients with onset at 0 - 4 years (55 %, P < 0.05), 0 - 9 years (46 %, P < 0.01) and 0 - 14 years (39 %, P < 0.01), but a decrease when age of onset was over 25 years (16 %, P < 0.05).

5.5.3. Total Number of Patients

Distribution of frequency was similar to that found in males: an increase in patients with onset at 0 - 9 years (45 %, P < 0.001) but a decrease when age of onset was over 25 years (16 %, P < 0.001).

5.6. Focal Sign

The correlation between age at onset of seizure and focal sign in EEG is analyzed. The high frequency of patients with focal

sign was found in both sexes to be associated with an age of
onset between 0 - 2 years (29 % for males and 30 % for females).
Thereafter, the frequency gradually decreased until the age at
onset of 35 years, when it increased.

The frequency was found to be enhanced in females with age at
onset of 35 years or more (30 %, $P < 0.05$) and in the total number of patients between the ages of 35 and 39 years (32 %, $P < 0.05$).

The minimum frequency was found in males with onset at ages 10 -
14 and 15 - 19 years and in females with age of onset between
10 - 14 years.

6. Age at Onset of Seizure and Familial Predisposition

The correlation between age of onset of seizure and familial
predisposition to epilepsy is shown in Table 35.

A higher frequency of familial predisposition to epilepsy was
observed in patients of both sexes with onset of seizure at an
early age. The increased frequency of familial predisposition
was observed in males with the age at onset of 0 - 14 years (16 %,
$P < 0.001$), in females 0 - 9 years (16 %, $P < 0.01$), and in total
patients aged 0 - 4 years (18 %, $P < 0.05$), 0 - 9 years (15 %,
$P < 0.05$), and 0 - 14 years (14 %, $P < 0.01$) than in those with
other age at onset of seizure. Decreased frequency was found in
males with onset of seizure at 20 or more years (3.5 %, $P < 0.01$)
and in the total patients (3.5 %, $P < 0.001$), when age at onset
was 20 or more years.

These findings correspond to the results reported in previous
studies indicating that early-onset epileptics might have a higher
incidence of familial predisposition (OUNSTED, 1952; BEAUSSART and
BEAUSSART-BOULENGE, 1969; GREGORIADES, 1972); conversely, late-
onset epileptics had a lower incidence of familial predisposition
(0 % in patients with onset after age 40 years: MAYER and
TRÜBESTEIN, 1968). These results may also correlate with type
of seizure and presence of exogenous factors.

Only 2 of our patients with a family history of epilepsy had
their first seizure after the age of 30 years. The mean age at
onset of seizure among patients with familial predisposition
to epilepsy was 13.7 ± S.E. 0.33 for males, 9.2 ± 0.97 for females, and 12.1 ± 0.20 years for all patients. Among patients
with no family predisposition, these figures were 19.8 ± 0.07,
17.7 ± 0.07, and 18.9 ± 0.03 years, respectively.

The difference was statistically significant in males ($t = 2.028$,
d.f. = 274, $P < 0.05$), in females ($t = 2.642$, d.f. = 188, $P < 0.01$), and in total patients ($t = 3.423$, d.f. = 464, $P < 0.001$).
Thus, male and female patients with familial predisposition to
epilepsy showed an earlier onset of seizure than male and female
patients with no familial predisposition.

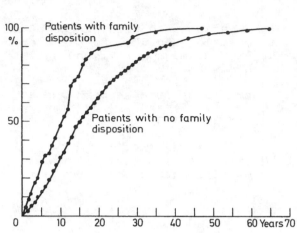

Fig. 8. Accumulative frequency of age at onset of seizure of patients with and without familial predisposition

The cumulative incidence of age at onset of seizure among patients with and those without familial predisposition is shown in Figure 8.

7. Age of Onset of Seizure and Exogenous Factors

As shown in Table 36, the frequency of patients with exogenous factors was higher in male patients with onset of 0 - 1 year and 20 - 39 years (P < 0.001) and in the total number of patients in these age ranges (P < 0.001) than in others. In female patients, the presence of exogenous factors was observed with a higher frequency in patients with an earlier onset; however, the difference was not statistically significant.

In previous studies, STÖGMANN and LORENZONI (1970) reported a high incidence of exogenous factors such as microcephaly and hydrocephaly among early-onset epileptics. SOMASUNDARAM et al. (1969) reported brain damage as a cause of seizure. Among late-onset epileptics, brain neoplasms as well as cerebrovascular lesions were frequently observed (WHITE et al., 1953; NIEDERMEYER, 1958; WOODCOCK and COSGROVE, 1964; MAYER and TRÜBESTEIN, 1968; CARNEY et al., 1969; BANCAUD et al., 1970; COURJON et al., 1970; BONDUELLE et al., 1970; VERCELLETTO and DELOBEL, 1970; FEUERSTEIN et al., 1970; KUHLO and SCHWARZ, 1971).

8. Evolution of Type of Seizure and Time of Occurrence

Patients with Pure Type of Seizure. In addition to a single clinical type of seizure, about half of our patients experienced additional types of seizure, as shown in Tables 22, 23, and 24, and in Figure 5. According to various types of seizure, a percentage of patients with a combined type has been shown: patients with A-GM (64 %), with S-GM (56 %), with D-GM (62 %), with absence PM (87 %), with myoclonic PM (88 %), with psychomotor

epilepsy (80 %), and with cortical epilepsy (55 %) (see Table 5).
An analysis of the kind of clinical association or combination
likely to appear has been made in Chapter III.12.

The frequency of patients with pure type (only one type of seizure) was lower in patients with absence PM (13 %, P < 0.001),
in those with myoclonic PM (12 %, P < 0.001), total petit mal
(16 %, P < 0.001), in those with awakening grand mal (36 %,
P < 0.001), and in patients with psychomotor epilepsy (20 %,
P < 0.001). The frequency was higher only in patients with occasional grand mal (45 %, P < 0.01), and in patients with grand
mal during sleep (44 %, P < 0.05).

A difference in frequency of patients with pure type of seizure
existed between male and female patients (54 % in male, 43 % in
female, P < 0.05). This frequency difference was due mainly to
the difference in total grand mal (51 % vs. 38 %, P < 0.05),
but was not significant in each type of grand mal.

Patients with Petit Mal and Grand Mal. Seventy-nine patients
(41 males and 38 females) were found to have petit mal in addition to grand mal. Combined grand•mal was mainly A-GM. These
patients were divided into three groups according to time of
occurrence of other types of seizure. The group of 32 patients
with petit mal followed by grand mal showed the highest frequency with age at onset of seizure between 6 and 7 years (median 7 years of age). This was 2 years later than in the group
of 16 patients with pure petit mal (4 - 5 years of age). The age
at onset of subsequent grand mal in these patients was highest
in frequency at age 14 - 15 years.

In the 12 patients who first developed grand mal, and subse-
quently petit mal, age at onset of seizure ranged from 7 months
to 20 years (median 10 years of age). The subsequent petit mal
frequently occurred at age 14 years.

Among 35 patients with a simultaneous occurrence of both petit
mal and grand mal, a peak of frequency at 8 - 9 years of age was
observed. This was 2 years later than in patients who had petit
mal followed by grand mal, and the 35 patients clearly showed
bimodal curves, as seen in Figure 9. Another peak of distribution
was seen at age 12 - 13 years.

These observations correspond to the authors' findings reported
in Chapter III, in which petit mal commonly occurred in the age
range of 6 - 10 years, and awakening grand mal between 9 - 15
years. Nevertheless some differences were observed in age at
onset of seizure in these 79 patients. Pure petit mal occurred
at a very early age; petit mal followed by grand mal occurred
at a slightly later age; and patients with both types occurring
at the same time had their first seizures at a rather late age.
This finding corresponds with the results observed by CURRIER
et al. (1963) and LIVINGSTON et al. (1965), who stated that
petit mal was apt to be combined with grand mal in patients
with a later onset.

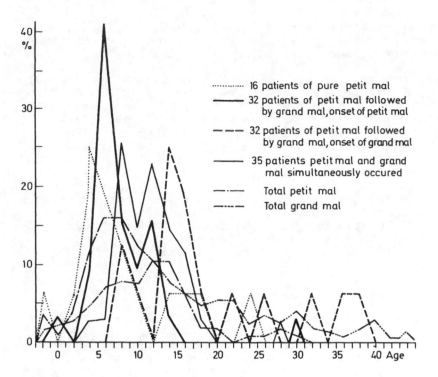

Fig. 9. Distribution by age at onset of seizure and evolution of type of seizure

In previous studies, clinical association between certain types of seizure has been shown. In some patients, petit mal was transformed into grand mal at puberty (GASTAUT, 1954), at 12 - 14 years of age (HERTOFT, 1963), or within 5 years of onset (GIBBERD, 1966). These findings were confirmed in this study. This age range, puberty, is critical for patients with epilepsy because many patients have their first seizure at this age. Also many petit mal patients in this age range develop grand mal as their second type of seizure. However, seizures of many petit mal patients were also found to stop at puberty (CURRIER et al., 1963; LIVINGSTON et al., 1965).

9. Early, Teen-Age, Middle-Age, and Late-Onset Epilepsy

Data are reported for four groups of patients divided according to age at onset of seizure, i.e., between 0 and 9 years (early onset), 10 - 19 years (teen-age onset), 20 - 39 years (middle-age onset) and 40+ years (late onset). Results are shown in Table 37.

With respect to type of seizure, patients with early onset revealed a higher frequency of awakening grand mal, absence petit mal (32 %, P < 0.001), and total petit mal (42 %, P < 0.001) than others.

The patients with teen-age onset showed a higher frequency of awakening grand mal (43 %, P < 0.001), and myocolonic petit mal (14 %, P < 0.001), but a decreased frequency of psychomotor epilepsy (18 %, P < 0.01), than did patients with onset within other age ranges.

The patients with middle-age onset indicated a lower frequency of awakening grand mal and a decreased frequency of absence petit mal (3 %, P < 0.001, together with late-onset patients), myoclonic petit mal (2 %, P < 0.001, together with late-onset patients), and of total petit mal (5 %, P < 0.001, together with late-onset patients).

The late-onset patients showed a decreased frequency of awakening grand mal (14 %, P < 0.05), absence, myoclonic, and total petit mal, but an increased frequency of grand mal during sleep (39 %, P < 0.01).

Data from previous studies may be summarized as follows. Patients with early onset of epilepsy (0 - 9 years of age) seemed to show a higher frequency of grand mal or petit mal and a lower incidence of cortical as well as psychomotor epilepsy, when compared with patients with onset at 10 - 15 years (GOMES LINS and FARIAS da SILVA, 1969). In early childhood, various types of seizure were observed according to age at onset (LENNOX and DAVIS, 1950; JANZ and MATTHES, 1955). Late-onset epileptics exhibited mainly grand mal, cortical epilepsy, or temporal lobe epilepsy (WHITE et al., 1953; FISCHER, 1959; MAYER and TRÜBESTEIN, 1968; FERNANDEZ SALAS et al., 1969; BONDUELLE et al., 1970; FEUERSTEIN et al., 1970; KUHLO and SCHWARZ, 1971; NIEDERMEYER, 1958). These results correspond to those reported in this study.

With regard to paroxysmal EEG abnormalities, basic EEG rhythm, familial predisposition to epilepsy, and exogenous factors, patients with early onset of seizure had a higher frequency of paroxysmal EEG abnormalities (71 %, P < 0.01), sp-w-c (28 %, P < 0.001, together with teen-age onset patients), abnormal EEG (56 %, P < 0.01), slow waves (52 %, P < 0.001), pathologic changes during hyperventilation (45 %, P < 0.001), and familial predisposition to epilepsy (15 %, P < 0.001, together with the teen-age group) than others.

Patients with teen-age onset showed similar but slightly milder symptoms than those observed in patients with early onset. Patients with middle-age onset revealed an intermediate pattern between the early-onset and late-onset groups. The late-onset patients showed inverse symptoms to those of the early-onset group: a low frequency of paroxysmal EEG abnormalities (39 %, P < 0.01); sp-w-c (5.6 %, P < 0.05); and no α-wave (P(Fisher) = 0.013). Slow waves (14 %, P < 0.01), pathologic changes during hyperventilation (14 %, P < 0.05), and familial predisposition were also decreased in incidence.

10. Summary

Characteristic findings concerning the correlation between patients with different ages at onset of seizure and (1) paroxysmal EEG abnormalities, (2) basic EEG rhythm, (3) familial predisposition to epilepsy, (4) the presence of exogenous factors, and (5) type of seizure are discussed in this chapter. Significant findings are summarized in Table 38.

In male patients, distribution by age at onset of seizure showed an initial peak at 0 - 1 year. Many patients with D-GM, psychomotor epilepsy, atypical sp-w-c, and exogenous factors were found to have their first onset of seizure at this age. However, the main peak in incidence was found at 10 - 13 years age.

In female patients, the initial peak was not observed. Instead, a bimodal curve was observed with the first peak found at 6 - 7 years of age (principally characteristic of those with absence PM) and the second peak at 12 - 13 years of age (principally characteristic of those with A-GM). The peak of the distribution in female patients occurred at an earlier age than in male patients.

Each type of seizure had its own characteristic distribution range with respect to age of onset. The frequency of paroxysmal EEG abnormalities, especially sp-w-c, was highest in those with a younger age of onset and decreased with increasing age of onset. Familial predisposition to epilepsy was more common in those patients with onset at an early age and this also decreased with age. Exogenous factors were frequently found in patients with onset at 0 - 1 year of age and in the middle-age group at onset (20 - 39 years).

The four groups of patients (early, teen-age, middle-age, and late-onset) showed characteristic findings in connection with each factor. Early as well as teen-age onset epileptics showed a higher frequency of A-GM, absence PM, myoclonic PM, paroxysmal EEG abnormalities, especially sp-w-c, high-voltage α-rhythm, slow waves, pathologic findings during hyperventilation, and familial predisposition to epilepsy. Conversely, a decreased frequency was found in patients with S-GM, D-GM, and psychomotor epilepsy, β-EEG, and low voltage EEG. Late-onset epileptics revealed characteristics inverse to those mentioned above. Middle-age-onset patients showed an intermediate pattern between the above-mentioned group.

The evolution of type of seizure and its occurrence was analyzed. Patients with PM followed by GM were found to have early onset at prepuberty, which was 2 years later than pure PM; their GM occurred at 12 - 13 years of age. Patients with simultaneous occurrence of PM and GM showed the latest onset at puberty.

V. Paroxysmal EEG Abnormalities

The authors took 3/s (typical) sp-w-c, atypical sp-w-c, sharp
and slow waves, spikes, temporal discharge, and sharp wave as
paroxysmal EEG patterns in the present study.

The correlation between paroxysmal EEG patterns and age, basic
EEG rhythm, familial predisposition to epilepsy, and exogenous
factors are shown in Table 39.

1. Incidence of Spike-and-Wave Complex

The incidence of sp-w-c among unselected epileptics has been reported by various authors to be between 5.5 - 25 %, the median
being 14.6 % (ROBINSON and OSTERHELD, 1947; CLARK and KNOTT,
1955; STRACKEE-KUIJER, 1957; ARIMA, 1959). These incidences were
apparently higher than those found among unselected neuropsychiatric patients (2 - 9.5 %, the median 7.2 % reported by SILVERMAN,
1954; LUNDERVOLD et al., 1959; TAKASE, 1960; DALBY, 1969).

The incidence of 3/s sp-w-c among unselected epileptics was found
to vary from 3.0 - 19.5 %, the median being 6.0 % (JASPER and
KERSCHMAN, 1941; FINLEY and DYNES, 1942; GIBBS et al., 1943;
CLARK and KNOTT, 1955; HAUGSTED and HÖNKE, 1956; STRACKEE-KUIJER,
1957; ARIMA, 1959). These incidences were higher than those found
among unselected neuropsychiatric patients (0.7 - 7.5 %, the median 1.1 % reported by SILVERMAN, 1954; LUNDERVOLD et al., 1959;
TAKASE, 1960; DALBY, 1969). A small percentage of neuropsychiatric patients was found among patients with sp-w-c at an incidence between 1.4 and 3.0 % (SILVERMAN, 1954; GOTO, 1957;
LUNDERVOLD et al., 1959; NIEDERMEYER, 1966; DALBY, 1969).

2. Paroxysmal EEG Abnormalities and Age

2.1. Male Patients

The frequency of paroxysmal EEG patterns was higher in 3/s sp-w-c
in patients with aged 10 - 34 years (6.6 %, P < 0.05); in atypical
sp-w-c in those aged 5 - 34 years (11 %, P < 0.05); total sp-w-c
in patients aged 5 - 34 years (17 %, P < 0.001); and in total
paroxysmal patterns in those aged 5 - 14 years (81 %, P < 0.05),
and 5 - 19 years (71 %, P < 0.01) than in those of other ages
(see Table 39). The distribution of paroxysmal EEG patterns by
age can be seen in Table 39 and Figure 10a. As indicated above,
the frequency of paroxysmal EEG patterns in patients aged 5 - 9
and 10 - 14 years was higher (81 %). After age 20 years, the frequencies were between 45 and 60 %. However, the frequency of total sp-w-c EEG abnormality was highest in patients aged 10 - 14
years (14 %) and thereafter decreased gradually with age, ap-
pearing again in a second peak at 25 - 34 years of age (15 %).

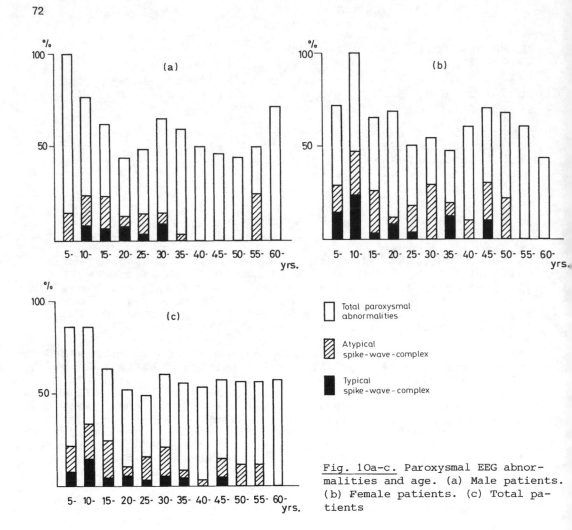

Fig. 10a-c. Paroxysmal EEG abnormalities and age. (a) Male patients.
(b) Female patients. (c) Total patients

2.2. Female Patients

There was an increased frequency of paroxysmal EEG patterns in
patients aged 5 - 14 years (92 %, P < 0.01). The distribution of
paroxysmal EEG patterns by age is shown in Table 39 and Figure
10b. At age 5 - 9 and 10 - 14 years there was a peak; during the
years between 25 and 39 the curve was concave, with another peak
seen at 45 - 54 years. In the distribution of sp-w-c EEG abnormality, the highest peak was observed at 10 - 14 years (47 %);
thereafter, it decreased rapidly with age.

2.3. Total Number of Patients

The distribution of paroxysmal EEG patterns by age was similar
to that found in male and female patients, as indicated in Table
39 and Figure 10c.

The frequency of paroxysmal EEG patterns was greater in patients
in the 5 - 14 year age group (86 %, P < 0.001) than in those in
other age groups. The observed frequency was higher in 3/s sp-w-c
in patients aged 5 - 24 years (8 %, P < 0.05); in atypical sp-w-c
at the age of 5 - 19 years (19 %, P < 0.01); and in those with
total sp-w-c at the age of 5 - 19 years (27 %, P < 0.001).

Corresponding observations by various authors have been presented
in previous studies. During repeated examination the frequency
of EEG abnormality was highest at age 0 - 9 years, and thereafter
decreased linearly with age (AJMONE MARSAN and ZIVIN, 1970).
ROBINSON and OSTERHELD (1947) found the highest frequency of
EEG abnormality, and of sp-w-c in patients aged 10 - 14 years
(40 %, P < 0.01, by the authors), thereafter decreasing with
age, with the decrease more pronounced concerning sp-w-c.
LUNDERVOLD et al. (1959) studied 363 patients with sp-w-c, con-
sisting of 13 % with 3/s sp-w-c, 33 % with atypical sp-w-c and
normal basic EEG rhythm, 41 % with atypical sp-w-c and abnormal
basic rhythm, and 14 % with focal sp-w-c. Younger patients showed
an increased frequency of typical sp-w-c (patients aged 0 - 20
years, 15 %, P < 0.05); atypical sp-w-c with abnormal basic
rhythm (patients aged 0 - 15 years, 48 %, P < 0.01) and focal
sp-w-c (patients aged 0 - 10 years, 20 %, P < 0.01); and the least
frequency of atypical sp-w-c with normal background (patients
aged 0 - 15 years, 21 %, P < 0.001) (statistical analysis was
made by the authors).

Several authors also reported the maximum distribution of sp-w-c
in patients aged 4 - 14 years (GOTO, 1957), in those aged 6 - 10
years (LUNDERVOLD et al., 1959), in those aged 10 - 15 years
(MORITA, 1960), and in those aged 5 - 14 years (DALBY, 1969).
LENNOX and DAVIS (1950) compared distribution of 200 patients
with 3/s and 200 patients 2/s sp-w-c by age, and found a marked
difference: an increased frequency between 1 and 4 years of age
among patients with 2/s sp-w-c; and, conversely, a high incidence
of patients with 3/s sp-w-c over 13 years of age. A similar distribution by age was also found by LUNDERVOLD et al. (1959);
the highest distribution of 3/s sp-w-c was seen in patients
aged 10 - 14 years and that of other types of sp-w-c, as well
as focal sp-w-c, was demonstrated in patients aged 5 - 9 years.

JANZ (1969) reported a correlation between age and frequency of
sp-w-c; that is, patients of 3 - 4 years are apt to reveal a
slower rate than 3/s, and those of 10 - 12 years a faster rate
than 3.5/s sp-w-c. HESS and NEUHAUS (1952) reported a close
electroclinical correlation between age and EEG as well as type
of seizure. However, GLASER and GOLUB (1955) found no difference
in frequencies of paroxysmal or focal abnormality in patients
with psychomotor epilepsy between children of 1.6 - 9 years and
patients of 10 - 16 years (66 % vs. 67 %).

As indicated in Table 2, younger patients showed the highest as
well as the most highly increased frequency of paroxysmal, sp-w-c,
and abnormal EEG patterns. These frequencies were found to be
decreased in adult patients and lowest in aged patients. Among
patients who suffered from head injury, schizophrenia, and psy-

chopathic personality, as well as in normal control subjects, the highest frequency of EEG abnormality was found in the youngest age group. The frequency thereafter was found to decrease linearly with age (YOSHII et al., 1970; HILL, 1952). However, SILVERMAN et al. (1955) found a higher incidence of EEG abnormality in aged normal subjects (60+ years of age) than in the younger control individuals (18 - 54 years of age). The incidence increased with age over 60 years. OTOMO and TSUBAKI (1966) reported a high frequency of EEG abnormality among aged subjects over 60 years of age (average 74 years, 54 % of 650 EEGs of 466 subjects). They also found an increase of EEG abnormality in normal subjects over age 60 (33 % in the age group 60 - 69, 41 % in 70 - 79, and 56 % in 80+ years).

The above-mentioned results might be correlated with cerebral maturation according to age: the decrease of incidence of slow waves, stabilizing of α-rhythm, and increasing tendency of seizure threshold. Type of seizures also affects the incidence of EEG abnormality.

2.4. Comparison Between Findings in Male and Female Patients

A similar distribution by age was seen in male and in female patients with regard to the frequency of paroxysmal EEG patterns. The differences were as follows: the frequency of paroxysmal EEG abnormality, especially sp-w-c, was increased in female over male patients (22 % vs. 12 %); this difference was found in those over 30 years (5.8 % vs. 20 %, P < 0.01). In males, there was a decrease. The individual paroxysmal potentials were counted and are shown in Tables 17 and 18. The most frequently observed paroxysmal potential was the sharp wave in both sexes. Seventy-six patients (16 %) showed sp-w-c; the frequency was greater in female than in male patients (22 % vs. 12 %, P < 0.01). In these potentials, 3/s sp-w-c, irregular sp-w-c, 3.5-5/s sp-w-c, and multiple sp-w-c were seen in 5 - 7 % of the cases. Only the difference in frequencies of 3.5-5/s sp-w-c, and multiple sp-w-c was significant (9.5 % for females and 2.5 % for males, 3.5-5/s sp-w-c, P < 0.01; 10 % for females and 5.4 % for males, multiple sp-w-c, P < 0.05; see Table 27). The sharp wave was found in 30 % and 28 %; and sharp and slow waves in 8.7 % of males and 6.8 % of females, respectively. Temporal discharge was observed in only 17 patients; 11 patients showed a clinical seizure during EEG examination. These were mostly of the petit mal type.

Female predominance was found in patients with 3/s sp-w-c (60 % female of 200 patients, LENNOX and DAVIS, 1950; 66 % female of 56 patients, GOTO, 1957); male predominance has been reported in slow sp-w-c (61 % male of 200 patients, LENNOX and DAVIS, 1950; 59 % male of 17 patients, GOTO, 1957), in irregular sp-w-c (56 % male of 57 patients, GOTO, 1957), and in multiple sp-w-c (63 % male of 19 patients, GOTO, 1957; 67 % male of 55 patients, HORI, 1959); almost the same distribution (105 males and 110 females) as reported by NIEDERMEYER (1966). The sex ratio reported in the total number of patients studied was nearly equal (GOTO, 1957; MORITA, 1960; TAKASE, 1960).

3. Paroxysmal EEG Abnormalities and Sex

As mentioned in Chapter II and in the preceding paragraph some differences between the sexes were observed in paroxysmal EEG patterns. For instance, female patients showed an increased frequency of atypical sp-w-c (16 % for females, 8 % for males, P < 0.01) and of total sp-w-c (22 % vs. 12 %, P < 0.01); they also showed a higher frequency of 3/s sp-w-c (6 % vs. 4 %). However, the frequency of paroxysmal EEG patterns was nearly the same (57 % vs. 63 %) for both sexes. When the frequency of paroxysmal EEG abnormalities in patients with each type of seizure was compared, the frequency of patients with 3.5-5/s sp-w-c as well as of multiple sp-w-c was higher in female than in male patients. Otherwise no significant differences were noted.

The observations in the present study correspond to those in previous studies.

4. Paroxysmal EEG Abnormalities and Type of Seizure

The correlation between type of seizure and paroxysmal EEG patterns is shown in Tables 14 and 15 and analyzed in Chapter III. This correlation is also reflected in Table 16.

Correlations between paroxysmal EEG abnormalities and types of seizure as reported in the literature are summarized in Table 40.

The patients with sp-w-c frequently developed petit mal (41 - 70 %, median 60 %) and grand mal (16 - 78 %, median 61 %). Other authors have reported a great variety in the incidence of both petit mal and grand mal. Our patients with sp-w-c also showed psychomotor, cortical, myoclonic, and akinetic types of seizures. Patients with 3/s sp-w-c frequently revealed petit mal (62 - 82 %, median 71 %), and, less frequently, grand mal (26 - 86 %, median 54 %). Patients with slow sp-w-c showed a higher frequency of grand mal than of petit mal; and myoclonic as well as akinetic seizures were often observed.

Patients with multiple sp-w-c showed a marked increase of grand mal (56 - 85 %, median 61 %), and, less frequently, petit mal (8 - 38 %, median 23 %, with wide variations). In addition, myoclonic as well as akinetic seizures were frequently observed (HORI, 1959; GOTO, 1957). JASPER and KERSCHMAN (1949) and later PENFIELD (1954) and JANZ and CHRISTIAN (1957) also reported that multiple sp-w-c is common in patients with myoclonic epilepsy. GIBBS and GIBBS (1952) reported that the frequent occurrence of multiple spikes during sleep in petit mal patients was attributable to a grand mal component. Contrary to the above and to GASTAUT's observations (1954), NIEDERMEYER (1966) failed to show a consistent association of paroxysmal abnormality with myoclonic manifestation. GOTO (1957) failed to find any affinity with respect to type of paroxysmal EEG activity and clinical seizure in general.

As analyzed in Chapter III.5, a study of contingent factors clearly revealed specific correlations between certain types of seizures and corresponding paroxysmal EEG abnormalities.

5. Paroxysmal EEG Abnormalities and Age at Onset of Seizure

The correlation between paroxysmal EEG patterns and age at onset of seizure is indicated in Tables 32 and 37. The analysis has been presented in Chapter IV. With respect to the correlation, several results have been reported in previous studies.

All patients with paroxysmal EEG abnormality showed an earlier onset of seizure than those without this abnormality. The frequency in total patients with age at onset under 14 years increased in paroxysmal EEG abnormality (67 %, P < 0.001), in 3/s sp-w-c (9.6 %, P < 0.001), in atypical sp-w-c (16 %, P < 0.01), and in total sp-w-c (25 %, P < 0.001) than in those with age at onset of 15+ years. Similar findings were observed in male and in female patients.

Distribution by age at onset of seizure in patients with sp-w-c was highest in those about 8 years old and thereafter decreased with age (GOTO, 1957). With respect to the type of paroxysmal EEG abnormalities, patients with 3/s sp-w-c showed a remarkably high frequency at age of onset of 5 - 12 years (60 %), thereafter decreasing rapidly (LENNOX and DAVIS, 1950). A similar distribution curve was also observed by GOTO (1957) and LUNDERVOLD et al. (1959).

An increased frequency of 2/s sp-w-c was observed in the age groups with onset of 0 - 1 and 0 - 4 years, when compared with those with 3/s sp-w-c (LENNOX and DAVIS, 1950). Distribution by age of onset of seizure in patients with 2/s sp-w-c was similar to that found in patients with atypical sp-w-c and focal sp-w-c (LUNDERVOLD et al., 1959). The increased frequency of 2/s sp-w-c in patients with age at onset in infancy or early childhood might be correlated with (1) a higher frequency of West and Lennox syndrome occurring in these patterns, (2) a greater tendency towards seizure, (3) liability to brain damage in this age range, and (4) electroclinical association between 2/s sp-w-c and West as well as Lennox syndrome.

The markedly high incidence of 3/s sp-w-c in patients with age at onset of 5 - 12 years might be correlated with (1) a higher frequency of petit mal occurring in these patients, (2) a greater tendency of seizure, especially for girls, (3) an endocrine disturbance at puberty for girls, and (4) electroclinical association between 3/s sp-w-c and petit mal.

There were a few patients with sp-w-c who first experienced onset of seizure after 20 or 30 years. LENNOX and DAVIS (1950) found only 2 patients (1 %) with 3/s sp-w-c and 3 patients (1.5 %) with 2/s sp-w-c whose age at onset was more than 19 years. When onset occurred after 26 years, LUNDERVOLD et al. (1959) failed to find any patients with 3/s sp-w-c; however, he noted 12 patients with

atypical sp-w-c (3.9 %). When onset occurred after age 20, GOTO
(1957) found only one patient with 3/s sp-w-c (1.6 %) and 9 patients with atypical sp-w-c (7.1 %).

In the present study, as shown in Chapter V.2 and Table 2, 23
patients (4.9 %) were revealed sp-w-c at ages over 30 years. The
characteristic findings in these patients are analyzed in Chapter V.16.

6. Paroxysmal EEG Abnormalities and α-EEG

The correlation between paroxysmal EEG patterns and basic EEG
rhythm is shown in Table 39.

In general, there was no close correlation between the distribution of patients with normal α, high voltage α, or no α-EEG and
the presence of paroxysmal EEG patterns. Nevertheless, there
was an increased number of patients with high voltage α or no
α-EEG among those with atypical sp-w-c in male (32 % vs. 15 %,
$P < 0.001$) and female patients (46 % vs. 25 %, $P < 0.05$) than
among those with no atypical sp-w-c. In the total number of patients, there was an increased incidence of high voltage α-EEG
in those with atypical sp-w-c (19 % or 10 of 52 patients, $P <
0.05$) and in patients with total sp-w-c (16 % or 15 of 96 pa-
tients, $P < 0.01$); and an increased incidence of normal α-rhythm
in the total number of patients with total sp-w-c (62 %, $P <
0.001$) and in those with atypical sp-w-c (60 %, $P < 0.001$). Pa-
tients with high-voltage α-EEG showed a tendency toward a higher
frequency of 3/s sp-w-c and of paroxysmal EEG patterns; however,
this was not statistically significant.

7. Paroxysmal EEG Abnormalities and β-EEG

There was no close correlation between paroxysmal EEG patterns
and β-EEG. A higher incidence of β-EEG was found in patients
with atypical sp-w-c (25 % or 13 of 52 patients) as well as in
those with total sp-w-c, but the difference was not statistically
significant.

8. Paroxysmal EEG Abnormalities and Slow Waves

A higher incidence of slow waves was found in the following instances: (1) in male patients with paroxysmal EEG abnormalities
(48 % or 76 of 157 patients, $P < 0.001$) and in those with atypical sp-w-c (59 % or 13 of 22 patients, $P < 0.05$); (2) in female
patients with paroxysmal EEG abnormalities (52 % or 62 of 119
patients, $P < 0.001$); (3) in the total number of patients with
paroxysmal EEG abnormalities (50 % or 138 of 276 patients, $P <
0.001$), with atypical sp-w-c (52 % or 27 of 52 patients, $P < 0.05$)
and with total sp-w-c (51 % or 39 of 76 patients, $P < 0.01$).

The incidence of very slow waves (θ - δ) was higher in female patients with paroxysmal EEG patterns (30 % or 36 of 119 patients, P < 0.01), in the total number of patients with total sp-w-c (28 % or 21 of 76 patients, P < 0.01), and in those with paroxysmal EEG abnormalities (20 % or 55 of 276 patients, P < 0.01).

9. Paroxysmal EEG Abnormalities and Low Voltage EEG

Four out of 13 patients with low voltage EEG revealed a paroxysmal EEG activity: two exhibited sharp and slow waves; the other two had only sharp waves. No patient showed sp-w-c or spike waves. The patients with low voltage EEG indicated a lower frequency of paroxysmal EEG activity than did the total number of patients (31 % vs. 3.4 %, P < 0.05).

10. Paroxysmal EEG Abnormalities and Pathologic Findings During Hyperventilation

Male patients with pathologic findings during hyperventilation showed a higher incidence of 3/s sp-w-c (13 %, P < 0.001), atypical sp-w-c (22 %, P < 0.001), total sp-w-c (35 %, P < 0.001), and of paroxysmal EEG abnormalities (89 %, P < 0.001) than did those with no pathologic findings during hyperventilation. In female patients with pathologic change during hyperventilation, a higher frequency was found in 3/s sp-w-c (8 %, P < 0.001), atypical sp-w-c (23 %, P < 0.001), total sp-w-c (31 %, P < 0.001) and in paroxysmal EEG abnormality (92 %, P < 0.001). In the total number of patients with pathologic change during hyperventilation, a higher frequency was also found in 3/s sp-w-c (15 %, P < 0.001), atypical sp-w-c (30 %, P < 0.001), total sp-w-c (45 %, P < 0.001), and paroxysmal EEG abnormality (90 %, P < 0.001).

11. Paroxysmal EEG Abnormalities and Focal Sign

An increased frequency of patients with focal sign was found in males with paroxysmal EEG abnormalities (75 %, P < 0.01), in females (82 %, P < 0.05), and in the total number of patients (78 %, P < 0.001). Patients with sp-w-c showed a lower frequency of focal sign in males (3 % or 1 of 34 patients, P < 0.05) and in the total number of patients (4 % or 3 of 76 patients, P < 0.01). The frequency of patients with focal sign in the total number of patients with atypical sp-w-c was also lower (6 % or 3 of 52 patients, P < 0.05). No patient with 3/s sp-w-c showed focal sign. HESS et al. (1970) reported the simultaneous occurrence of temporal focal and generalized paroxysmal EEG abnormalities.

12. Paroxysmal EEG Abnormalities and Familial Predisposition

Patients with paroxysmal EEG activity showed a higher frequency
of patients with family history of epilepsy (positive family
disposition); however, this was not statistically significant
in males, females, or in the total number of patients. On the
other hand, patients with EEG sp-w-c abnormality showed an increased frequency of familial predisposition in males (29 % or
10 of 34 patients, P < 0.001) and in the total number of patients
(21 % or 16 of 76 patients, P < 0.001) than did those with no
sp-w-c; however, in females it was not statistically significant
(14 % or 6 of 42 patients).

There was a higher frequency of familial predisposition to epilepsy in male and in total patients with paroxysmal EEG abnormalities (67 %, P < 0.05; 70 %, P < 0.05, respectively). In female patients, similar findings were obtained; however, the tendency was not statistically significant. Only one patient with
temporal discharge had a positive familial predisposition to
epilepsy. In previously reported studies the incidence of a positive familial predisposition among patients with sp-w-c ranged
from 20 - 50 % (HILL, 1952; GOTO, 1957; LUNDERVOLD et al., 1959;
DALBY, 1969), the median being 28 %. The figure in our study was
21 %. The following is a comparison of previously reported data
with data from the present study. Incidence varied with respect
to the type of paroxysmal EEG abnormalities: for 3/s sp-w-c,
17 - 34 % (median 27 %), 17 % in this study; for slow sp-w-c,
9 - 48 % (median 27 %), 20 % in this study; for multiple sp-w-c,
4 - 26 % (median 15 %), 30 % in this study; for focal sp-w-c 8 -
24 % (median 13 %); and for 3.5-5/s sp-w-c, 24 % in this study.

As previously mentioned (Chapter III), a family history of epilepsy is of little etiologic significance unless the family com-
position and degree of relationship between members are known.
However, the present authors did compare previously reported
frequencies with respect to the type of paroxysmal EEG abnormalities. The patients with 3/s sp-w-c reported by GOTO (1957)
showed an increased frequency of a positive familial predisposition when compared with control patients (27 % vs. 15 %, P < 0.05,
authors' calculation); the frequency with a positive family history in patients with total sp-w-c (20 % or 27 of 136 patients)
was also higher than in control patients (15 % or 76 of 504 patients); however, the difference was not statistically significant.

Patients with 3/s sp-w-c showed a higher incidence of familial
predisposition than those with 2/s sp-w-c; however, the difference
was not significant (34 % vs. 27 %, LENNOX and DAVIS, 1950; 27 %
vs. 17 %, GOTO, 1957). GABOR and AJMONE MARSAN (1969) found a
higher incidence of positive familial predisposition in 35 patients with bilateral focal sp-w-c (11 %) than in 67 patients
with unilateral focal sp-w-c (6 %), but the difference was also
not significant. Our patients with paroxysmal EEG abnormalities
under the age of 19 years showed a higher frequency of familial
predisposition (P < 0.05). This finding corresponds to that reported by ROBERT and KARBOWSKI (1971). Patients with sp-w-c EEG
over 40 years had a higher frequency of familial predisposition

(43 %, or 3 of 7 patients) than those under the age of 39 years
(19 %, or 13 of 69 patients); however, the difference was not
statistically significant.

As reported in this study, HOCKADAY and WHITTY (1969) also found
that patients with familial predisposition showed a higher frequency of EEG abnormality.

13. Paroxysmal EEG Abnormalities and Exogenous Factors

In patients with and those without paroxysmal EEG activity, no
difference was found in frequencies of the presence of exogenous
factors. However, patients with 3/s sp-w-c and those with atypical sp-w-c had a lower frequency of the presence of exogenous
factors than other patients. The frequency of the presence of
exogenous factors was higher in patients with temporal discharge;
however, the difference was not statistically significant. In
general, patients with sp-w-c were found to have a lower frequency of the presence of exogenous factors. AJMONE MARSAN and
ZIVIN (1970) reported that exogenous factors do not play a role
in the etiology of EEG abnormalities in epileptics. Other authors,
however, have reported such factors as a high incidence of breech
delivery (CHURCHILL, 1959) and low birth weight (HORI, 1959) as
significant etiologic factors. EEG sp-w-c has been shown to occur
in patients with hypothalamic pituitary tumor (SCHERMAN and
ABRAHAM, 1963), head traumatism (NIEDERMEYER, 1966), and cerebral lesions (TÜRKEL and JASPER, 1952).

A significantly higher frequency in the presence of exogenous
factors among patients with 2/s or slow sp-w-c (42 %) compared
with patients with 3/s sp-w-c (4 %) has been indicated by
LENNOX and DAVIS (1950), and also by SILVERMAN (1954), CLARK
and KNOTT (1955), and ISHIKURO (1957). In this study, patients
with sp-w-c, especially those with 3/s sp-w-c, with 3.5-5/s
sp-w-c as well as with multiple sp-w-c revealed a lower frequency
of the presence of exogenous factors than did those with atypical
sp-w-c. The difference found by LUNDERVOLD et al. (1959) was not
significant, since the incidence in patients with 3/s sp-w-c
(30 %) was apparently high compared to 43 % in patients with
other types of sp-w-c. Among patients with multiple sp-w-c, the
incidence observed varied widely from 7 to 75 % (NIEDERMEYER,
1966; GOTO, 1957; HORI, 1959). HORI (1959) reported a higher
frequency of exogenous factors among patients under the age of
14 when compared with those over 15 years of age.

14. Patients With and Without Paroxysmal EEG Abnormalities

The results of a comparative analysis of patients with and without paroxysmal EEG abnormalities are shown in Table 41. Compared
with 190 patients with no paroxysmal EEG abnormalities, 276 patients with paroxysmal EEG abnormalities had a higher frequency
of early (0 - 9 years) onset (33 % vs. 20 %, P < 0.01) and a lower
frequency of late onset of seizure (12 % vs. 5 %, P < 0.01); a

higher frequency of awakening grand mal (38 % vs. 22 %), of absence (18 % vs. 10 %), myoclonic (10 % vs. 3 %), and total petit mal (30 % vs. 13 %), very slow θ - δ waves (20 % vs. 11 %), pathologic changes during hyperventilation (46 % vs. 7 %), and focal sign in EEG (20 % vs. 8 %). A lower frequency of grand mal during sleep (15 % vs. 25 %) and of diffuse grand mal (16 % vs. 21 %) was also observed (results of statistical analysis were reported previously).

15. Patients With Typical, Atypical, and Total Spike-and-Wave Complex (Table 42)

Seventy-six patients with total sp-w-c showed a higher frequency of awakening grand mal, of Lennox syndrome, of absence, of myoclonic, and of total petit mal, of high-voltage α-rhythm, of slow waves, of pathologic changes during hyperventilation, and of focal sign in EEG.

Patients with typical or atypical sp-w-c were compared separately. Twenty-four patients with typical sp-w-c revealed a higher frequency in age at onset of 0 - 14 years and in awakening grand mal; however, there was a lower frequency of β-EEG and no α-wave was observed. The only statistically significant difference was in those with absence (54 % vs. 25 %, P < 0.05) and in those with total petit mal (79 % vs. 56 %, P < 0.05).

16. Patients With Spike-and-Wave Complex at Age Over 30 Years (Table 42)

As previously shown in Chapter V.2 and Table 2, patients with sp-w-c were found mainly at younger ages. In this study, however, 23 patients (4.9 % of total patients) over the age of 30 demonstrated sp-w-c. Six of them revealed typical sp-w-c and 17 showed atypical sp-w-c, together representing 30 % of all patients in the study with sp-w-c. BECK (1971) reported that 9.8 % of patients with sp-w-c were over 30 years of age. The sex ratio in these patients was 16 females (8.4 %) to 7 males (2.5 %, P < 0.01). As shown in Table 42, 23 patients with sp-w-c over the age of 30 showed a higher frequency at early onset (0 - 9 years, 48 %, P < 0.01), a higher frequency of awakening grand mal (70 %, P < 0.001), of absence petit mal (35 %, P < 0.01), and of myoclonic petit mal (22 %, P < 0.01), whereas grand mal during sleep (no patients, P(Fisher) = 0.0067), diffuse grand mal (9 %), and psychomotor epilepsy (9 %, P(Fisher) = 0.040) were lower in frequency. Six patients showed β-EEG and 4 patients exhibited high voltage α-rhythm; however, no patients were found with low voltage EEG or focal sign in EEG (P(Fisher) = 0.019). An increase in frequency was found in patients with pathologic changes during hyperventilation (83 %, P < 0.001) and in familial predispositon to epilepsy (30 %, P < 0.001).

As previously mentioned in Chapter V.2, and indicated in Table 42, compared with 390 patients with no sp-w-c 76 patients with

total sp-w-c showed a younger age at onset of seizure, a higher
frequency in three types of seizure — A-GM, absence PM, and myoclonic PM — and, conversely, a lower frequency in three other
types of seizure — S-GM, D-GM, and psychomotor epilepsy. A higher
incidence was observed in patients with very slow waves, high-
voltage α-rhythm, pathologic changes during hyperventilation,
and with familial predisposition to epilepsy. Frequency of patients with focal sign in EEG was lower.

Similar but more pronounced findings were observed in patients
over 30 years of age with sp-w-c. When 23 patients over 30 years
of age with sp-w-c were compared with 253 patients with other
types of paroxysmal EEG abnormalities, differences were significant in frequency in female patients (70 % vs. 41 %, $P < 0.01$),
in early onset of 0 - 9 years, in A-GM (70 % vs. 35 %, $P < 0.01$),
S-GM (0 % vs. 16 %, $P(Fisher) = 0.021$), absence PM (35 % vs. 17 %,
$P < 0.001$), myoclonic PM (22 % vs. 9 %, $P < 0.05$), pathologic
changes during hyperventilation (57 % vs. 43 %, $P < 0.001$), focal
sign in EEG (22 % vs. 0 %, $P(Fisher) = 0.004$), and in familial
predisposition (30 % vs. 10 %, $P < 0.01$), as indicated in Table 42.

17. Paroxysmal EEG Evolution

LESNY (1971) followed up 11 patients with hypsarrhythmia at infancy or in early childhood. A few years later, he found 6 patients with slow sp-w-c (55 %), and one patient each with generalized sinus wave and bifrontal synchronous slow wave; 3 patients showed no change. CAVAZZUTI et al. (1971) reported EEG
evolution from hypsarrhythmia to focal slow sp-w-c abnormality.

Paroxysmal EEG evolution of 2/s sp-w-c to or through 3/s sp-w-c
to multiple sp-w-c has been reported by several authors (GIBBS
and GIBBS, 1952; PAAL, 1957; HESS, 1958; BAMBERGER and MATTHES,
1959). JANZ (1969) described the frequency change of a rate
slower than 3/s at age 3 - 4 years to faster than 3.5/s sp-w-c
at age 10 - 12 years.

18. Summary

Paroxysmal EEG abnormalities, especially sp-w-c, were frequently
found in young patients as well as in patients with early onset
of seizure; incidence decreased with age. In female patients,
total sp-w-c, atypical, 3.5-5/s, and multiple sp-w-c was higher
in frequency than in males. Certain paroxysmal EEG patterns
showed close correlations with certain types of seizures, e.g.,
3/s sp-w-c and absence PM as well as A-GM; and temporal discharge
and psychomotor epilepsy. For these correlations, the authors
have made use of the coefficient of contingency analysis. Some
correlations between paroxysmal EEG abnormality and basic EEG
rhythm were seen. Patients with sp-w-c showed an increased incidence of high voltage α, β, slow waves, and pathologic findings
during hyperventilation. On the other hand, a decreased frequency
of low voltage EEG as well as focal sign in EEG was seen. Patients

with sp-w-c EEG abnormality were found to show an increased frequency of familial predisposition to epilepsy. Patients with sp-w-c indicated a lower frequency of the presence of exogenous factors.

VI. Basic EEG Rhythm

1. α-EEG

The correlation between α-EEG and age, EEG findings, familial predisposition, and exogenous factors are analyzed.

The correlation between α-EEG and sex, type of seizure, age at onset of seizure, and paroxysmal EEG patterns have previously been analyzed.

1.1. α-EEG and Age

Among the total number of patients, the incidence of normal α-EEG was lowest at 5 - 9 years (64 %), increasing gradually thereafter, and reaching 100 % at over age 65. The frequency of normal α-EEG at the age of 5 - 14 years (66 % or 37 of 56 patients, $P < 0.05$), and also at the age of 5 - 19 years (71 %, $P < 0.05$), was lower compared with those with other age groups. Conversely, in the 5 - 14 year age group, the incidence of high voltage α-rhythm was higher (20 %, $P < 0.05$).

Similar findings were observed in male patients: the incidence of high-voltage α-rhythm was higher at 5 - 14 years (19 %, $P < 0.01$), but that of normal α-EEG was lower in the same age range (66 %, $P < 0.01$). These tendencies were also found in female patients; however, they are not statistically significant.

PETERSEN and EEG OLOFSSON (1971) observed the increase of α-frequency linearly with age in normal children. In patients with myoclonic petit mal, CHRISTIAN (1968) found good α-rhythm at 10 - 11 c/s. The frequency in patients with normal α-rhythm was lowest at the age of 5 - 14 years, and thereafter increased with age.

1.2. α-EEG and Pathologic Findings During Hyperventilation

Patients with high-voltage α-EEG showed a higher frequency of pathologic findings during hyperventilation; however, this was not statistically significant.

1.3. α-EEG and Focal Sign

No close correlation between α-rhythm and focal sign was found.

1.4. α-EEG and Familial Predisposition

Patients with high voltage α-rhythm or no α-rhythm, compared with those with normal α-rhythm, showed an increased frequency of familial predisposition to epilepsy in males (20 % vs. 9 %, P < 0.01), and in the total number of patients (16 % vs. 8 %, P < 0.05).

1.5. α-EEG and Exogenous Factors

No close correlation was found between α-rhythm and the presence of exogenous factors.

2. β-EEG

The correlation between β-EEG and age, EEG findings, familial predisposition and exogenous factors are analyzed. The correlations between β-EEG and sex, type of seizure, age at onset of seizure, and paroxysmal EEG activities were previously analyzed.

Among epileptic patients, the presence of β-waves clearly increased in incidence compared with a normal control group (very fast wave: 8.9 % vs. 0.4 %, fast wave: 17 % vs. 6.2 %; GIBBS et al., 1943). This increase in very fast wave was also observed among epileptic patients under 20 years of age (2.6 %).

2.1. β-EEG and Age

Patients with β-EEG ranged from 9 - 75+ years. Female patients showed an increased incidence of β-EEG compared with male patients (23 % vs. 14 %, P < 0.05), as indicated in Chapter II. There was an increased incidence of β-EEG in the 10 - 39 year age group in females (27 %, P < 0.05) as well as in the total number of patients (20 %, P < 0.01). This increase was also observed in male patients; however, it was not statistically significant. After the age of 40 years, the inicidence of β-EEG decreased in males.

According to GIBBS et al. (1943) the incidence of β-wave was higher in adults than in persons under 20 years of age (very fast wave, 8.9 % vs. 2.6 %; fast wave, 17 % vs. 5.7 %).

An increased incidence of β-EEG was observed in female patients over 35 years and especially in those over 45 (VOGEL and GÖTZE, 1962). In the present study, β-EEG was found predominantly in female patients. This increase, however, was not found in aged female patients, but in the age group of 10 - 39 years. Male patients in this age range also showed a higher incidence but the difference was not significant.

2.2. β-EEG and Pathologic Findings During Hyperventilation

Patients with pathologic findings during hyperventilation showed
a lower incidence of β-EEG; however, this was not statistically
significant.

2.3. β-EEG and Focal Sign

Patients with focal sign showed a lower incidence of β-EEG; however, this was not statistically significant.

2.4. β-EEG and Familial Predisposition

Patients with familial predisposition to epilepsy showed a higher
incidence of β-EEG in males, in females, and in the total number
of patients; however, these differences were not statistically
significant.

2.5. β-EEG and Exogenous Factors

No correlation was found between β-EEG and the presence of exogenous factors.

VOGEL and GÖTZE (1962) found the incidence of β-EEG to be 5.5 %
for males and 12 % for female patients. According to the authors'
calculations the difference between these figures was significant.
In patients with seizure, VOGEL and GÖTZE reported an incidence
of 8.5 % for males and 13 % for females; this difference was not
significant. A predominantly higher incidence of β-EEG among females than among male patients was observed not only among epileptics but also among all patients examined at their EEG labo-
ratory. This tendency has also been found by others (JUNG, 1952;
SMITH, 1954).

In correlating the incidence of β-EEG with sex and age, no differences are reported in males; however, an increased incidence
at 35+ and especially at 45+ years has been noted for female
patients (VOGEL and GÖTZE, 1962). VOGEL (1958) found a small
increase of β-EEG among normal twin girls, but GARSCHE (1956)
failed to find any sex difference in incidence. MUNDY-CASTLE
(1951) also failed to find any age effect.

3. Slow Waves

Slow waves as defined by the authors in this study represent an
excess or predominance of θ wave or δ wave.

According to GIBBS et al. (1943) the incidence of slow waves
was higher in adult epileptics (16 % for θ wave, 13 % for δ wave)

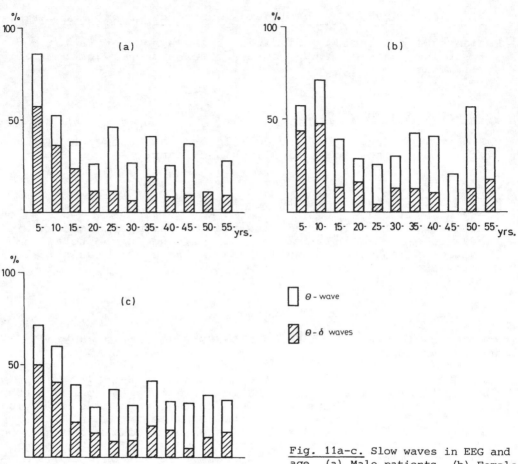

Fig. 11a-c. Slow waves in EEG and age. (a) Male patients. (b) Female patients. (c) Total patients

and in child epileptics (18 % for θ wave) than in controls (7.6 % for θ wave). The correlations between slow waves and sex, type of seizure, the age at onset of seizure, and paroxysmal EEG abnormalities have been analyzed above.

The correlations between slow waves and age, other EEG findings, familial predisposition, and exogenous factors are analyzed.

3.1. Slow Waves and Age

Distribution of patients with slow waves by age is shown in Figure 11a-c. In male patients, the incidence of slow waves was higher in the 5 - 9 year age group (86 %, P < 0.05); in the total patients in the 5 - 14 year age group (62 %, P < 0.001); and in female patients in the 5 - 14 year age group (67 %, P < 0.01) than in other age groups.

The incidence of θ-waves was seen constantly with age in about
20 - 30 % in males and in the total patients. Conversely, in female patients, one could see the increasing frequency of θ waves
with age. A decreasing frequency of slow waves with age was apparently due to a decreasing tendency of θ - δ waves with age in
males, in females, and in the total patients.

Among normal children between 0 and 15 years of age, EEG OLOFSSON
(1971) and PETERSEN and EEG OLOFSSON (1971) observed the highest
incidence of slow waves at 5 - 7 years of age, decreasing after
that age span. HILL (1952) also analyzed correlation between age
and θ-dominant EEG. Nonepileptic subjects in the 0 - 10 year age
group showed a higher incidence (25/409, 5.0 %) than those in
the 11 - 18 year age group (14/559, 2.5 %). The difference was
significant (P < 0.01). At 18 years or older, the incidence was
still lower (1/147, 0.7 %). Among epileptic children and ado-
lescents, a similar finding was observed: The incidence of θ-
dominant EEG in the 0 - 10 year age group (22/190, 12 %) was
higher than in the 11 - 18 year age group (11/201, 5.5 %, P < 0.05).

Among healthy aged subjects, some authors have reported a lower
incidence of θ-EEG than in young normals (MUNDY-CASTLE, 1951;
YOSHII, 1971). A significant difference was found between aged
(average 75 years) and young (average 22 years) healthy persons
(28 % vs. 65 %, P < 0.001).

3.2. Slow Waves and Pathologic Findings During Hyperventilation

Compared with patients with no slow waves, in patients with slow
waves an increased frequency of pathologic findings during hyperventilation was found in males (38 % vs. 26 %, P < 0.05) and in
the total patients (37 % vs. 27 %, P < 0.05); however, in female
patients the frequency was not statistically significant. Marked
correlations were also found between θ - δ waves and pathologic
findings during hyperventilation in females (48 % vs. 28 %,
P < 0.05) and in the total patients (41 % vs. 28 %, P < 0.05);
however, in male patients this was not statistically significant.

3.3. Slow Waves and Focal Sign

A comparison of 75 patients with very slow (θ - δ) waves with
those with no θ - δ waves showed an increased frequency of focal
sign in females (28 % vs. 12 %, P < 0.05) and in the total patients (25 % vs. 14 %, P < 0.01).

3.4. Slow Waves and Familial Predisposition

There was no correlation between the incidence of slow waves
and familial predisposition to epilepsy.

3.5. Slow Waves and Exogenous Factors

A higher frequency in the presence of exogenous factors was found in patients with θ - δ waves than in those with no θ - δ waves, but it was not statistically significant.

PETERSEN and EEG OLOFSSON (1971) reported that slow waves are always related to age (maximum in the 5 - 7 year age group) and to sex (more frequent among female subjects). According to HILL (1952), θ-dominant EEG was found more frequently among epileptic patients (8.4 %) than among nonepileptic patients (4.0 %). The difference was significant (P < 0.01, calculated by the authors). The incidence of epileptic patients with θ-dominant EEG was highest at age 0 - 5 years, thereafter decreasing with age. A similar distribution by age was also found among nonepileptic patients. Among healthy subjects over 50 years of age, YOSHII (1971) found an increasing tendency toward slow waves.

The increase of slow waves was frequently observed not only among epileptics but also in patients with some neurologic diseases, such as Huntington's chorea (VOGEL et al., 1961a), mental retardation, encephalopathies (FUJIMORI et al., 1958), etc.

No other correlations can be made due to lack of data in previous studies.

4. Low Voltage EEG

The correlation between low voltage EEG and sex, type of seizure, age at onset of seizure, paroxysmal EEG abnormalities, α-EEG, β-EEG, and slow wave dominant EEG have previously been analyzed.

The correlation between low voltage EEG and age, other EEG findings, familial predisposition, and exogenous factors are analyzed.

According to GIBBS et al. (1943), the frequency of low voltage EEG was not increased, but was decreased in adults (2.6 %). No epileptic children showed this EEG finding.

4.1. Low Voltage EEG and Age

In the present study there were no patients with low voltage EEG in the 5 - 19 year age group. All patients with low voltage EEG were found only in the 20 - 49 year age group (P(Fisher) = 0.0035).

Among the aged subjects, the frequency of low voltage (flat) EEG was irrelevant to age or to the presence of neurologic signs (OTOMO and TSUBAKI, 1966). In this study, this type of EEG was found only in the adult age group.

4.2. Low Voltage EEG and Pathologic Findings During Hyperventilation

Only two patients with low voltage EEG showed pathologic findings during hyperventilation.

4.3. Low Voltage EEG and Focal Sign

No patients with low voltage EEG showed focal sign.

4.4. Low Voltage EEG and Familial Predisposition

No correlation between low voltage EEG and the presence of familial predisposition to epilepsy was found.

4.5. Low Voltage EEG and Exogenous Factors

Patients with low voltage EEG seemed to have a tendency toward the presence of exogenous factors, but this was not statistically significant.

ADAMS (1959) concluded that there is no correlation between low voltage EEG and epilepsy, because he could find no patient with low voltage EEG among 665 epileptics. However, VOGEL (1962) failed to confirm this conclusion when he observed the same incidence of epilepsy in patients with this kind of EEG and in patients without it.

The correlation between this EEG finding and some neurologic diseases such as Huntington's chorea (VOGEL et al., 1961a) and head traumatism (GÖTZE, 1957) was studied. MEYER-MICKELEIT (1953) observed no significant increase of low voltage EEG in patients with head trauma. OTOMO and TSUBAKI (1966) found no difference in the frequency of low voltage EEG pattern among neurologically normal and abnormal aged subjects.

5. Correlated Findings in Patients With Various Types of Basic EEG Rhythm

Some characteristic findings in patients with different basic EEG rhythms are shown in Table 43.

5.1. Patients with High Voltage α-EEG

High voltage α-EEG occurred with an increased frequency in female patients (60 %, P < 0.01), in those with awakening grand mal (45 %, P < 0.05), and in patients with sp-w-c (32 %, P < 0.01); it was observed, but with decreased frequency, in patients with

grand mal during sleep and diffuse grand mal (23 %, P < 0.05),
when compared with those with other type of basic EEG rhythms.

5.2. Patients With Normal α-Wave

Normal α-waves were found more frequently in females than in
male patients (37 %, P < 0.01).

5.3. Patients With β-EEG

Compared with patients with no β-EEG, patients with β-EEG revealed an increased incidence of myoclonic petit mal (17 %,
P < 0.001), total petit mal (35 %, P < 0.01), but a decrease of
grand mal during sleep (11 %, P < 0.05).

5.4. Patients With Slow Waves

In a comparison of patients with and without slow waves, it was
observed that patients with slow waves showed an increased frequency with age at onset in the 0 - 9 year age group (40 %, P <
0.001), and in those with paroxysmal EEG abnormalities (82 %,
P < 0.001) and sp-w-c (23 %, P < 0.01). The frequency was lower
in the age group with onset over 40 years (3 %, P < 0.01).

5.5. Patients with Low Voltage EEG

These patients showed an increased frequency with age of onset
between 20 - 39 years (77 %, P < 0.001), and in those with occasional grand mal (62 %, P < 0.001), but a decrease in those
with awakening grand mal (P(Fisher) = 0.048), total PM (P(Fisher)
= 0.033), paroxysmal EEG abnormalities (31 %, P < 0.05), and at
age of onset between 0 - 19 years (23 %, P < 0.01).

5.6. Comparison Between Patients With Various Basic EEG Rhythms

Patients with high-voltage α-wave and those with β-EEG showed
very similar findings, as shown in Table 43. There was no marked
difference in any category.

In comparing patients with high voltage α-wave and those with
slow waves, the former revealed a higher frequency among female
patients (60 % vs. 42 %, P < 0.05) and patients with sp-w-c (not
significant). Cortical epilepsy and paroxysmal EEG abnormalities
(68 % vs. 82 %, P < 0.05) were observed less frequently in the
former.

In comparing patients with high voltage α-wave and with those
with low voltage EEG, the latter showed a lower frequency in
female patients, in those with age at onset of 0 - 19 years (66 %

vs. 23 %, P < 0.05), in patients with awakening grand mal (45 %
vs. 8 %, P < 0.05), in total petit mal (30 % vs. 0 %, P(Fisher)
= 0.020), in patients with paroxysmal EEG abnormalities (68 % vs.
31 %, P < 0.05), and in sp-w-c (32 % vs. 0 %, P(Fisher) = 0.014).
The frequency increased inversely in patients with occasional
grand mal (13 % vs. 62 %, P < 0.001) as well as in those with
slow waves (30 % vs. 77 %, P < 0.001).

Patients with high voltage α-wave were also compared with those
with normal α-rhythm. The patients with high voltage α-wave
showed an increased frequency in female patients (60 % vs. 37 %,
P < 0.01), in patients with awakening grand mal (45 % vs. 30 %,
P < 0.05), in those with paroxysmal EEG abnormalities, and in
sp-w-c (32 % vs. 13 %, P < 0.001). The frequency decreased inversely in those with grand mal during sleep, cortical epilepsy
(0 % vs. 10 %, P(Fisher) = 0.011), and slow waves.

In a comparison between patients with β-EEG and those with slow
waves, there was a difference in patients with grand mal during
sleep (11 % vs. 21 %, P < 0.05), total petit mal (35 % vs. 24 %,
P < 0.05), and in those with paroxysmal EEG abnormalities (62 %
vs. 82 %, P < 0.001).

In a comparison between patients with β-EEG and those with low-
voltage EEG, there was a difference in the age group with onset
between 0 and 19 years (70 % vs. 23 %, P < 0.01), in those with
awakening grand mal (37 % vs. 8 %, P(Fisher) = 0.031), occasional
grand mal (15 % vs. 62 %, P < 0.001), total petit mal (35 % vs.
0 %, P(Fisher) = 0.0068), paroxysmal EEG abnormalities (62 % vs.
31 %, P(Fisher) = 0.037), sp-w-c (not significant), and in those
with slow waves (26 % vs. 77 %, P < 0.01).

Patients with β-EEG were compared with those with normal α-ryhthm.
In patients with β-EEG there was an increased frequency of females (53 % vs. 37 %, P < 0.01), in those with awakening grand
mal, myoclonic petit mal (17 % vs. 7 %, P < 0.01), and in total
petit mal (35 % vs. 21 %, P < 0.05), whereas the frequency of
patients with grand mal during sleep was lower (11 % vs. 20 %).

In a comparison between patients with slow waves and those with
low voltage EEG, there was a difference with onset between 0 and
19 years (73 % vs. 23 %, P < 0.001), in those with awakening
grand mal, occasional grand mal (17 % vs. 62 %, P < 0.001), total
petit mal (24 % vs. 0 %, P(Fisher) = 0.035), paroxysmal EEG abnormalities (82 % vs. 31 %, P < 0.001), and sp-w-c (23 % vs. 0 %,
P(Fisher) = 0.039).

Patients with slow waves were compared with those with normal
α-rhythm. The difference was found in those with paroxysmal EEG
abnormalities (82 % vs. 57 %, P < 0.001), sp-w-c (23 % vs. 13 %,
P < 0.01), and in those with the age of onset of 0 - 9 years (40 %
vs. 26 %, P < 0.01).

Patients with low voltage EEG were compared with patients with
normal α-wave. The former showed a decreased frequency with age
at onset between 0 and 19 years (23 % vs. 61 %, P < 0.05), in

patients with awakening grand mal (not significant), absence
petit mal, total PM (P(Fisher) = 0.048), paroxysmal EEG abnormalities, sp-w-c, and focal sign. Patients with low voltage EEG
also showed an increased frequency of patients with occasional
grand mal (62 % vs. 16 %, P < 0.001) and slow waves (77 % vs.
32 %, P < 0.01).

6. Pathologic Findings During Hyperventilation

Correlations between pathologic findings during hyperventilation,
sex, type of seizure, age at onset of seizure, paroxysmal EEG
abnormalities, and basic EEG rhythms have been analyzed previously.

Correlations between pathologic findings during hyperventilation
and age, other EEG findings, familial predisposition, and exogenous factors are analyzed.

6.1. Pathologic Findings During Hyperventilation and Age

The frequency of pathologic findings during hyperventilation was
highest in patients aged 5 - 9 years (79 %) and decreased gradually thereafter. The frequency in the 5 - 14-year age group was
higher in males (47 %, P < 0.05) than in females (65 %, P < 0.001)
and in the total number of patients (55 %, P < 0.001) than in
those in other age groups. On the other hand, the frequency decreased in patients over 35 years of age (17 %, P < 0.001).

The frequency of pathologic findings during hyperventilation
was highest in the 5 - 9-year age group; thereafter, it was found
to decrease linearly with age. This might be correlated with the
finding of θ-dominant EEG at this young age and with maturation
of brain.

6.2. Pathologic Changes During Hyperventilation and Focal Sign

No correlation was found between the presence of focal EEG sign
and pathologic findings during hyperventilation.

6.3. Pathologic Findings During Hyperventilation and Familial
Predisposition

A higher frequency of positive familial predisposition to epilepsy was found in patients with pathologic findings during hyperventilation; however, it was not statistically significant.

6.4. Pathologic Findings During Hyperventilation and Exogenous
Factors

Patients with pathologic findings during hyperventilation showed
an increased frequency in the presence of exogenous factors (18 %
vs. 11 %, P < 0.05).

Hyperventilation is a well-known method of provocation. The effect was greater in certain types of seizure such as Lennox syndrome (KRUSE, 1968), absence petit mal (JASPER and KERSCHMAN,
1941; HESS, 1958; LENNOX and LENNOX, 1960; LOISEAU et al., 1963),
myoclonic petit mal (JANZ and CHRISTIAN, 1957), and awakening
grand mal (CHRISTIAN, 1961). A considerable difference in the
effectiveness of hyperventilation in provoking awakening grand
mal compared with grand mal during sleep was observed (53 % vs.
14 %: CHRISTIAN, 1961). On the other hand, sleep activation was
more effective in patients with grand mal during sleep than in
patients with awakening grand mal (GÄNSHIRT and VETTER, 1961;
CHRISTIAN, 1961). The above correlations between type of seizure
and effectiveness of hyperventilation correspond with the results
in the present study as described in Chapter III. For patients
with psychomotor epilepsy, activation during sleep was more effective than hyperventilation (CHRISTIAN, 1968). Patients with
cortical epilepsy showed only slight response to hyperventilation,
as reported by JANZ (1969), and others; GABOR and AJMONE MARSAN
(1969) observed that patients with focal and bilateral synchronous epileptic discharge showed a greater response than those
with an unilateral focus without bilateral involvement.

7. Focal Sign

The correlations have already been analyzed with respect to the
presence of focal sign and sex, type of seizure, age at onset of
seizure, paroxysmal EEG abnormalities, α-EEG, β-EEG, slow waves
and low voltage EEG, and pathologic findings during hyperventilation.

Correlations between the presence of focal sign and age, familial
predisposition and exogenous factors are analyzed below.

7.1. Focal Sign and Age

Distribution of patients with focal sign by age was higher in
male patients of 30 – 44 years of age (24 %, P < 0.01), and in
female patients of 10 – 24 years of age (22 %, P < 0.05) than in
those in other age groups.

In male patients a higher or increased frequency was found in
the age ranges of 5 – 14 and 30 – 44 years. The difference of distribution in the two sexes might be attributed to a different
pathogenesis. In female patients, the higher frequency was seen
in the 10 – 24- and 50 – 64-year age groups.

Aged individuals were apt to have focal abnormality in the temporal area (HUGHES, 1967), and θ - δ focus (YOSHII et al., 1970).
Both references reported that a temporal lobe focus increased
linearly with age. On the other hand, focal abnormality was frequently observed among children (GIBBS and GIBBS, 1952; NIEDERMEYER
1957). With respect to the localization of focal abnormality by
age, LUNDERVOLD et al. (1959) frequently found temporal, parietal,
and occipital regions among younger patients (0 - 15 years of age),

and temporal, frontal, and parietal regions among adults. A relatively high frequency of focal abnormality was found among epileptic children (JERAS, 1970). KRUSE (1968) found 30 % focal abnormality among children who suffered from Lennox syndrome.

In the present study, the authors have failed to indicate any age correlation; a higher frequency of focal abnormality was found to exist only in male patients of 5 - 14 years of age. This might be correlated with the increase of organic change of the brain in patients with earlier onset.

7.2. Focal Sign and Familial Predisposition

No correlations was found between patients with focal sign and the presence of a positive familial predisposition to epilepsy.

7.3. Focal Sign and Exogenous Factors

Male patients with exogenous factors seemed to show an increased frequency of focal sign (33 % vs. 12 %, P < 0.001) than those with no exogenous factors. Similar findings were found in the total number of patients (32 % vs. 13 %, P < 0.001). In female patients, the increase was not statistically significant.

Previous reports showed no consistent distribution pattern by age or age at onset of seizure. This might be reflected by sampling methods. HUGHES (1967) found many patients with temporal foci at the age of 30 - 39 years and found another peak during adolescence.

LUNDERVOLD et al. (1959) observed a high frequency of focal abnormality among children with petit mal and sp-w-c. The number of patients with temporal focus increased with age (HUGHES, 1967), and aged patients were apt to have focal change (θ, δ-focus, YOSHII, 1971). With respect to localization of EEG focal abnormality, younger patients aged under 14 years were apt to show this focal change in the temporal, parietal, and occipital areas, whereas older patients aged 15+ years showed the abnormality in the temporal and frontal areas only. Among patients over 50 years of age, YOSHII (1971) found focal abnormality mostly in the temporal area. Patients with focal sp-w-c showed cortical seizures in 84 % of all cases (LUNDERVOLD et al., 1959).

A male predominance was seen among epileptic children with focal abnormality (56 % male vs. 44 % female: RICCI and SCARINCI, 1963). However, the sex ratio in the total patients under study must also be considered.

7.4. Patients With Focal EEG Abnormality on the Left or Right Side (Table 44)

Seventy-two patients with focal EEG abnormality were divided into two groups with respect to presence of EEG abnormality on the left or the right side. Among patients with focal abnormality on both sides, the more marked side of abnormality was considered.

More than 71 % of patients had left-sided abnormality. They showed a higher frequency of (1) early onset of seizures (0 - 9 years), (2) abnormality at the temporal area, (3) grand mal during sleep or psychomotor epilepsy, and (4) slow EEG waves. In addition, this group also showed a lower frequency of diffuse and occasional grand mal, paroxysmal EEG abnormalities, and the presence of exogenous factors. Difference in frequencies of diffuse grand mal (16 % vs. 38 %, P < 0.05), grand mal during sleep (28 % vs. 5 %, P(Fisher) = 0.026) and occasional grand mal (8 % vs. 33 %, P < 0.05) were statistically significant. Many patients with A-GM studied by BEYER and JOVANOVIC (1966) showed focal sign more on the left than on the right side (7.5 % vs. 2.5 %).

7.5. Patients With Focal EEG Abnormality at the Temporal or Extratemporal Area (Table 44)

Seventy-two patients were divided into two groups according to the area of focal EEG abnormality. Fifty-four patients (75 %) were found with temporal area abnormality and 18 (25 %) with the abnormality in the extratemporal area (3 frontal, 4 central/pre-central, 2 parietal, 6 occipital and 3 hemishperical).

Fifty-four patients with temporal focus showed a higher frequency of (1) grand mal during sleep or psychomotor epilepsy, (2) slow waves, and (3) familial predisposition to epilepsy. The difference was statistically significant in patients with grand mal during sleep (28 % vs. 0 %, P(Fisher) = 0.012) and in those with psychomotor epilepsy (59 % vs. 22 %, P < 0.05). These patients showed a lower frequency of cortical epilepsy (13 % vs. 33 %) and the presence of exogenous factors (17 % vs. 56 %, P < 0.01).

Extratemporal focus was more common in males: such patients also showed the reverse of findings exhibited by patients with temporal focus.

8. Summary

The number with normal α-rhythm was small in the younger patients, in the patients with younger age at onset of seizure, and in female patients. High voltage α-rhythm was frequently found in patients with (1) awakening GM, Lennox syndrome, absence PM, and with myoclonic PM, (2) paroxysmal as well as sp-w-c EEG, and (3) familial predisposition. On the other hand, the frequency was decreased in patients with S-GM, D-GM, and cortical epilepsy.

β-EEG was found increased in the 10 - 39-year age group, in those with age of onset of seizure within 5 - 19 years, in female over male patients, and when myoclonic PM, absence PM, sp-w-c, and familial predisposition to epilepsy were present.

Patients with slow waves were found more often among those of younger age and with younger age at onset, and in those with A-GM, myoclonic PM, and cortical epilepsy, as well as in paroxysmal and sp-w-c EEG, and with exogenous factors.

Patients with low voltage EEG were found only among adult patients. None of them exhibited sp-w-c. This type of EEG increased in patients with occasional GM and with cortical epilepsy, while it decreased in those with A-GM, Lennox syndrome, and with absence PM.

Patients with pathologic findings during hyperventilation were commonly found with A-GM and with absence PM, whereas the frequency decreased among those with S-GM and with D-GM. Many of them showed typical as well as atypical sp-w-c and also familial predisposition to epilepsy.

Patients with focal sign in the EEG were frequently found among those with psychomotor and with cortical epilepsy, and they showed an increased frequency of the presence of exogenous factors. Focal sign was seldom found in patients with A-GM, absence PM, or in patients with sp-w-c.

In the present study, focal abnormality in the EEG was found predominantly on the left side, and at the temporal area. The influence of the localization of focal abnormality, whether on the left or right side, temporal or other areas, was analyzed.

VII. Familial Predisposition

The correlation between the presence of familial predisposition to epilepsy and sex, type of seizure, age at onset of seizure, and EEG findings have been analyzed above. Of the 55 epileptic relatives identified, 16 were females, 22 males, and 17 of unknown sex.

The correlation between the presence of familial predisposition to epilepsy and age, and exogenous factors are analyzed.

1. Familial Predisposition[1] and Age

In patients with familial predisposition to epilepsy, an increased frequency was found in male patients of the 10 - 24-year age group than in those of other age groups (19 % vs. 5.5 %, P < 0.001) and in the total patients of the 10 - 19-year age group than in those of other age groups (20 % vs. 7 %, P < 0.001). These findings

---

[1]This information was not valid if the size of the family and the number and relationship of relatives were not defined. Familial predisposition in the present study refers to patients with at least one relative who suffered from epileptic seizure.

may be correlated with age at onset of seizure and also with type of seizure.

Epileptic children may have a higher frequency of family history of epilepsy than adult epileptics. This may also correlate with type of seizures. In general, patients who suffered from Lennox syndrome or absence petit mal showed a higher frequency of family history (42 %, BUENO et al., 1970; 44 %, CURRIER et al., 1963). RODRIGO LONDONO (1969) reported the highest frequency of 64 % among 500 epileptic children.

Among aged epileptics, the frequency of familial predisposition decreased inversely; the relative importance of exogenous factors such as brain tumor, cerebrovascular disease, and consumption of alcohol has been suggested by CARNEY et al. (1969), and GÄNSHIRT (1970).

2. Familial Predisposition and Exogenous Factors

Forty-six patients with familial predisposition to epilepsy revealed a decreased frequency of the presence of exogenous factors (only 1 patient) compared with those with no familial predisposition (2.2 % vs. 11 %, P < 0.05).

In general, as found in the present study, certain types of seizures, such as West and Lennox syndromes, are known to be frequently caused by exogenous factors. Patients with these syndromes are frequently found to have peri- or postnatal brain damage. Brain tumor or cerebrovascular lesion was also a common cause among late-onset epileptics, mostly with the cortical or grand mal type of seizure. On the other hand, prepuberty or teen-age-onset epileptics frequently showed familial predisposition to epilepsy but showed infrequently the presence of exogenous factors. The main types of seizures in this age group were awakening grand mal, absence PM, and myoclonic petit mal.

DALBY (1969) analyzed the incidence of epilepsy among relatives according to the proband's brain damage. Among 576 relatives of the brain-damaged group, 5.4 % were epileptic; the same incidence was found in the non-brain-damaged group (5.3 % or 49 out of 902 relatives). JANZ (1969) noticed a difference of familial predisposition to epilepsy between patients with cortical epilepsy with known etiology (1.3 %) and those without it (6.9 %). CURRIER et al. (1963) found a tendency toward an increased incidence of pure petit mal among patients with familial predisposition. Conversely, GIBBERD (1966) reported a tendency toward more grand mal association among petit mal patients with family history of epilepsy.

3. Patients With and Without Familial Predisposition

Table 45 shows a comparison of two groups of our patients divided according to the presence or absence of familial predisposition to epilepsy.

Compared with patients with no familial predisposition, patients
with familial predisposition showed an increased frequency of
age at onset between 0 and 9 years (41 % vs. 26 %, P < 0.05),
but a decreased frequency of age at onset at 20+ years (13 % vs.
40 %, P < 0.01).

The mean age at onset of seizure among patients with familial
predisposition was 12.1 years, and among those without familial
predisposition it was 18.9 years. The difference was statistically significant (t = 3.432, P < 0.001). The difference was
also confirmed in male (13.6 vs. 19.8 years, t = 2.028, P < 0.05)
as well as female patients (9.2 vs. 17.7 years, t = 2.642,
P < 0.01).

Patients with familial predisposition had an increased frequency
of absence (33 % vs. 13 %, P < 0.001) and total petit mal (41 %
vs. 21 %, P < 0.01). On the other hand, a lower frequency of
total grand mal and of psychomotor epilepsy was observed. An increased frequency of patients with sp-w-c (35 % vs. 14 %, P <
0.001) and abnormal EEG (59 % vs. 43 %, P < 0.05) were noted;
however, a decreased frequency of the presence of exogenous factors (2.2 % vs. 14 %, P < 0.05) was observed.

4. Similarity and Dissimilarity of Type of Seizure Between Proband and Epileptic Relatives

Epileptic relatives of patients with petit mal studied by MATTHES
and WEBER (1968) were found to have frequently a similar type
of petit mal seizure. Other authors have observed a greater frequency of grand mal than petit mal (CURRIER et al., 1963; GIBBERD,
1966; DALBY, 1969). THIERFELDER (1953) reported a similar type
of seizure among the probands with grand mal and their epileptic
family members.

Few observations regarding those relationships were obtained in
the present study. The authors plan to publish elsewhere clinical
and genetic studies related to epilepsy based on a larger patient
population than reported herein.

5. Summary

Compared with patients with no familial predisposition, patients
with familial predisposition to epilepsy showed an increased
frequency of earlier onset, absence PM, sp-w-c, and abnormal
EEG. On the other hand, the frequency was lower in those with
GM and with psychomotor epilepsy. Only one patient had familial
predisposition and exogenous factors.

Analysis of the familial occurrence of epilepsy indicates that
there is some degree of similarity in the type of seizure seen
in members of the same family but such frequencies should be
statistically analyzed in a larger sample.

VIII. Exogenous Factors

The correlation between the presence of exogenous factors and sex, type of seizure, age at onset of seizure, EEG findings, and familial predisposition to epilepsy have been analyzed previously.

The correlation between the presence of exogenous factors and age is analyzed.

1. Exogenous Factors and Age

Distribution of patients with exogenous factors by age was higher at age 30 - 49 years in males (28 %, P < 0.001) and in the total patients (20 %, P < 0.01), but decreased at the age of 50+ years in total patients (2.4 %, P < 0.05). In the 5 - 9-year age group the frequency of the presence of exogenous factors was higher in both sexes; however, it was not statistically significant.

The importance of exogenous factors among children as well as among aged epileptics has been noted by several authors (e.g., in West syndrome, CHARLTON and MELLINGER, 1970; STÖGMAN and LORENZONI, 1970; in Lennox syndrome, SCHNEIDER et al., 1970; and in aged patients, NIEDERMEYER, 1958).

HORI (1959) found a significant difference between the frequency of the presence of exogenous factors in children and in adults (84 % vs. 56 %, P < 0.05, calculated by the authors).

In the present study, the authors have indicated the increased frequency of familial predisposition among young epileptics and, simultaneously, the decreased frequency of exogenous factors. Inversely, among aged patients, there was an increased frequency of exogenous factors but a decreased frequency in familial predisposition. These observations correspond with previous findings in the above-mentioned references..The kinds of exogenous factors typical of young and aged patients were quite different. In the former, the authors frequently found peri- and postnatal brain damage or meningocerebral infection; whereas, as indicated in previous reports, in aged patients, head traumatism, brain tumor, and cerebrovascular lesion were more common.

2. Patients With and Without Exogenous Factors

Table 45 shows a comparison of two groups of our patients divided according to the presence or absence of exogenous factors.

Exogenous factors showed a decreased frequency of occurrence in female than in male patients, and among those with teen-age onset, awakening grand mal, grand mal during sleep, absence and total petit mal, and with familial predisposition. An increased frequency was found in patients of onset of 20 - 39 years, and in those with cortical epilepsy and with focal sign in EEG. The results of statistical analysis have been noted previously. Inverse findings were found in those patients with no exogenous factors.

Among patients with exogenous factors, the frequency distribution in grand mal observed in the present study corresponds with the results reported by JANZ (1953); that is, a lower frequency in patients with awakening GM and S-GM, and a higher frequency in those with diffuse grand mal.

Babies with low birth weight showed a markedly increased frequency of EEG abnormality compared to controls (AUCKLAND et al., 1969). According to STÖGMANN and LORENZONI (1970), patients who suffered from West syndrome and those with brain damage showed (1) earlier onset, (2) seizure type of Blitz- and Salaam-Krämpfen, (3) a neuropsychiatric complication, (4) a combination with grand mal, (5) lower frequency of family history, (6) EEG hypsarrhythmia, and (7) poor prognosis. On the contrary, patients with no brain damage showed (1) later onset, (2) a type of Nick-Krämpfen, (3) no neuropsychiatric complication, (4) a combination with Lennox syndrome, (5) higher frequency of familial predisposition, (6) EEG general paroxysm, and (7) good prognosis.

Patients with idiopathic epilepsy showed a higher frequency of EEG abnormality than did those with symptomatic epilepsy; however, the frequency of sp-w-c was not different in the two groups (27 % vs. 22 %: ROBINSON and OSTERHELD, 1947). CHURCHILL (1959) found a high frequency of breech delivery among epileptic patients (15 %) compared with that in the general population (3.5 %). Patients with diffusely abnormal EEG showed a higher frequency of breech delivery (20 %) than did those with localized EEG abnormality (2.8 %). Also, there was an increased frequency of breech delivery among patients with petit mal (40 %) and those with sp-w-c EEG (30 %) compared with patients with grand mal or other types (11 %).

3. Summary

The frequency of exogenous factors was found predominantly among male patients, increasing with age 30 - 49 years, age at onset of seizure of 0 - 1 and 20 - 39 years, and in patients with cortical epilepsy. Conversely, there was a decrease at teen-age-onset patients and in patients with A-GM, S-GM, and with absence PM.

IX. Conclusions

This study reports data from 466 nonselected epileptic patients of the Department of Neurology, University of Heidelberg. Data were analyzed multidimentionally from the following viewpoints: age, sex, age at onset of seizure, type of seizure, paroxysmal EEG abnormalities, basic EEG rhythm, familial predisposition to epilepsy, and exogenous factors. Although some of the correlations found in the present study were also studied by previous authors, this is the first known multidimensional analysis of a large group of nonselected patients.

1. Age-correlated factors were analyzed in Chapter I. Young, adult, and aged patients revealed typically different correlations. Compared to other age groups, patients under 19 years (26 % of the total number of patients) showed a higher frequency of awakening grand mal (A-GM, 36 %), absence petit mal (PM) (22 %), paroxysmal EEG abnormalities (74 %), sp-w-c (27 %), slow wave dominant EEG (50 %), pathologic findings during hyperventilation (42 %), and familial predisposition to epilepsy (18 %). On the other hand, a lower frequency of patients with grand mal during sleep (S-GM, 16 %), diffuse grand mal (D-GM, 12 %), low-voltage EEG (0 %), and exogenous factors (12 %) was observed in these patients. Inverse correlations were seeen in patients over 50 years (9 % of the total patients), i.e., a lower frequency was found in patients with A-GM (17 %), absence PM (7 %), myoclonic PM (0 %), cortical epilepsy (0 %), paroxysmal EEG abnormalities (56 %), sp-w-c (7 %), slow waves (32 %), pathologic changes during hyperventilation (17 %), familial predisposition to epilepsy (5 %), and the presence of exogenous factors (2 %). S-GM (37 %) and psychomotor epilepsy (44 %) was increased in frequency in aged patients. Adult patients between 20 and 49 years (65 % of the total patients) were found to have results intermediate to those of the above two age groups.

2. Correlations between sex and other factors were analyzed in Chapter II. Forty-one percent of our patients were female. Compared to male patients, female patients indicated a younger age distribution, earlier onset of seizure in general, and an increased frequency of total PM (27 % for females vs. 20 % for males), absence PM (18 % vs. 13 %), combined type of seizure (57 % vs. 46 %), atypical sp-w-c (16 % vs. 8 %), 3.5-5/s sp-w-c (10 % vs. 3 %), multiple sp-w-c (10 % vs. 5 %), and epileptic abnormal EEG (23 % vs. 13 %). Females showed a decreased frequency of cortical epilepsy (6 % vs. 9 %). With respect to basic EEG rhythm, female patients showed an increased frequency of high voltage α-rhythm (15 % vs. 7 % for males) and β-waves (23 % vs. 14 %). The frequency of familial predisposition to epilepsy (8 % vs. 11 %) as well as the presence of exogenous factors (6 % vs. 17 %) was higher in male patients.

3. Patients with each type of seizure were found to have individual characteristics regarding age at onset, and presence of paroxysmal EEG abnormalities, basic EEG rhythm, familial predisposition to epilepsy, and exogenous factors. Early, teen-age, middle-age, and late-onset patients showed different characteristic correlations with these factors. In many correlations, early- and late-onset epileptics were dissimilar. Several factors, such as type of seizure and EEG, were found to be clearly age-correlated. Coefficient contingency analyses distinguished between positive as well as negative associations among certain types of seizures and certain types of paroxysmal EEG abnormalities (Chapter III).

Patients with certain types of seizure were compared with those
with other types of seizure. If the difference was significant
the words increase or decrease were used. Characteristic findings
for patients with each type of seizure were as follows:

a) Awakening grand mal (84 male and 63 female patients) was found
   mostly in patients 10 - 39 years of age (85 %) and in the 6 -
   22-year age group at onset of seizure (78 %). A higher frequency was observed in patients with paroxysmal EEG abnormalities (71 %), including atypical sp-w-c (20 %), multiple sp-w-c
   (16 %), typical sp-w-c (12 %), and in 3.5-5/s sp-w-c (10 %).
   A higher frequency was observed in patients with high voltage
   α-rhythm (14 %), β-waves (20 %), pathologic findings during
   hyperventilation (42 %), and with familial predisposition to
   epilepsy (11 %), whereas the frequency of focal sign in EEG
   (7 %) as well as the presence of exogenous factors (8 %) was
   decreased.

b) Grand mal during sleep (53 male and 36 female patients) demonstrated an increased frequency in the age group over 45
   years (24 %) and in those whose age at onset was over 35 years
   (23 %). Patients with paroxysmal abnormalities were decreased
   in frequency (46 %); only one patient showed atypical sp-w-c
   (1 %), and there was neither typical nor multiple sp-w-c. A
   decreased frequency was found in patients with high voltage
   α-rhythm (4 %), β-waves (10 %), pathologic changes during
   hyperventilation (17 %), and with familial predisposition to
   epilepsy (7 %); the frequency of patients with focal sign in
   EEG (17 %) was increased. These findings were quite opposite
   to those found in patients with A-GM, and a very different
   clinical association pattern in both types of seizure was
   confirmed in association analysis.

c) Diffuse grand mal (50 male and 32 female patients). An increased frequency was observed in patients over 35 years
   (38 %), and in patients 0 - 4 years at onset of seizure (18 %).
   A decreased frequency of patients with paroxysmal EEG abnormalities (52 %), total sp-w-c (7 %), high voltage α-rhythm
   (9 %), pathologic changes during hyperventilation (24 %), and
   with familial predisposition to epilepsy (7 %) was also observed. There was a higher frequency of patients with focal
   sign in EEG (20 %) and with exogenous factors (16 %). Different features to patients with A-GM were found, but there
   were some similar findings to patients with S-GM.

d) Occasional grand mal (45 male and 31 female patients). No
   characteristic findings were observed.

e) West syndrome and Lennox syndrome. The authors could draw no
   definite conclusions because of the small number of patients
   (only 3 patients with West syndrome and 5 patients with
   Lennox syndrome).

f) Absence petit mal or pyknoleptic petit mal (35 male and 35
   female patients). Absence PM occurred with an increased frequency in females (50 %), in the 5 - 24-year age group (83 %),
   in those with age at onset of 5 - 17 years (83 %), and in those

with paroxysmal EEG abnormalities (73 %), including typical
sp-w-c (19 %), atypical sp-w-c (19 %), multiple sp-w-c (19 %),
and 3.5-5/s sp-w-c (11 %). Incidence among those with basic
EEG rhythm, high voltage α-rhythm (13 %), β-waves (21 %), and
pathologic changes during hyperventilation (51 %) was also
increased. Conversely, incidence was decreased in those with
focal sign (6 %) and low voltage EEG (O %). The highest frequency of patients with family history (21 %) and those with
the lowest frequency of the presence of exogenous factors (3 %)
among all types of seizure was shown in the present study.
There were some similar findings to those found in patients
with A-GM. Association analysis indicated a close correlation
between absence petit mal and awakening grand mal.

g) Myoclonic petit mal or impulsive petit mal (19 male and 16 female patients). All patients were in the 10 - 39-year age group.
A higher frequency was seen in those patients with age at onset at 10 - 16 years (71 %), and in those with paroxysmal EEG
abnormalities (83 %), including atypical sp-w-c (30 %), multiple sp-w-c (17 %), 3/s sp-w-c (17 %), β-waves (40 %), and in
those with pathologic changes during hyperventilation (51 %),
and familial predisposition to epilepsy (11 %). Low voltage
EEG was not observed; and focal sign in EEG was observed only
in 6 % of patients while the presence of exogenous factors was
found in 11 %. These unusual findings observed in patients with
myoclonic petit mal were also observed to some degree in patients with absence PM or A-GM. Association analysis confirmed
a close correlation among these syndromes.

h) Psychomotor epilepsy (65 male and 54 female patients). Patients
with psychomotor epilepsy were widely distributed by age. The
age at onset of seizure was most frequent at 0 - 5 years (21 %)
and 20 - 29 years (25 %). Patients with paroxysmal EEG abnormalities were low in frequency, e.g., typical sp-w-c (2 %)
and atypical sp-w-c (6 %), whereas the increase in isolated
temporal discharge (10 %) was significant. Focal, temporal,
or extratemporal nonspecific EEG abnormality (30 %) was also
higher. These characteristic findings were quite different
from those found in patients with A-GM or in those with absence or myoclonic PM. Association analysis, however, indicated the similarity of some findings in patients with grand
mal during sleep and those with diffuse grand mal.

i) Cortical epilepsy (29 male and 11 female patients). Less marked
findings were observed in patients with this type of seizure.
Male preponderance (73 %) and the increase of patients with
exogenous factors (33 %) was shown. Association analysis was
negatively correlated to other types of seizures.

The correlations between clinical type of seizure and paroxysmal EEG abnormality were studied and the results observed are
as follows:

A close correlation was observed between awakening grand mal
and presence of typical, atypical, 2-2.5/s, 3.5-5/s, and multiple
sp-w-c; between Lennox syndrome and the presence of atypical
and slow sp-w-c; between absence petit mal and the presence of

typical, atypical, 3.5-5/s, and multiple sp-w-c; between myoclonic petit mal and the presence of typical, multiple, and atypical sp-w-c; between psychomotor epilepsy and the presence of focal EEG abnormalities. In patients with D-GM and with S-GM, paroxysmal EEG abnormalities were low in frequency.

Clinical association between types of seizures in the same individuals was analyzed by the coefficient contingency analyses. A positive association was found between A-GM and absence PM, and A-GM and myoclonic PM. A less conclusive association was found between psychomotor epilepsy and S-GM, and between absence PM and myoclonic PM. Between other types, S-GM, and D-GM, and psychomotor and cortical epilepsy, there were negative associations only. Cortical epilepsy had no positive correlation with any other types of seizure.

With respect to the observations reported in Chapter III, patients with A-GM, with absence PM, and with myoclonic PM were found to have similar patterns of correlations. Other types of seizure — S-GM, D-GM, psychomotor epilepsy, and cortical epilepsy — showed patterns different from those found in the above-mentioned three types.

4. Characteristic findings in this study concerning the correlation between age at onset of seizure and (1) paroxysmal EEG activity, (2) basic EEG rhythm, (3) familial predisposition to epilepsy, (4) exogenous factors, and (5) type of seizure are indicated in Chapter IV. The significant findings were as follows:

Male patients revealed an initial peak at 0 - 1 year, which includes many patients with diffuse grand mal and psychomotor epilepsy and those with atypical sp-w-c and the presence of exogenous factors. The main peak was found at 10 - 13 years of age. In female patients, the initial peak was not observed. The distribution was bimodal, the first peak being found at 6 - 7 years of age, and included mainly patients with absence petit mal; the second peak was found at 12 - 13 years of age and included mainly patients with awakening grand mal. Female patients reached the peak of the highest distribution at a younger age than did male patients.

Patients with each type of seizure had characteristic distribution with respect to age range of onset of seizure.

The frequency of paroxysmal EEG abnormalities, especially of sp-w-c abnormality, was highest in patients with early onset and decreased with age. Familial predisposition was more common in those with early onset, and decreased with age. Exogenous factors were frequently found in patients with very early onset, in the 0 - 1-year age group (25 %) as well as in patients with onset during 20 - 39 years (21 %).

The four groups of patients (early, teen-age, middle-age, and late onset) showed characteristic findings in connection with each factor. Early- as well as teen-age-onset epileptics showed a higher frequency of patients with awakening grand mal(33 % for early-, 43 % for teen-age-onset patients); absence petit mal (32 %, 15 %); myoclonic petit mal (8 %, 14 %); paroxysmal EEG

abnormalities (71 %, 59 %), especially sp-w-c (28 %, 20 %), high
voltage α-rhythm (12 %, 10 %), and slow waves (52 %, 35 %), pathologic findings during hyperventilation (45 %, 32 %), and familial
predisposition to epilepsy (15 %, 13 %). Conversely, a decreased
frequency was found in patients with grand mal during sleep,
diffuse grand mal, psychomotor epilepsy, β-waves, and with low
voltage EEG. Late-onset epileptics revealed inverse findings to
those mentioned above. Middle-age-onset patients showed an intermediate pattern between those with early or teen-age onset and
those with late onset.

The evolution of the type of seizure and its occurrence was
analyzed. In patients with petit mal followed by grand mal, petit
mal occurred at prepuberty, and grand mal more frequently occurred at 12 - 13 years of age. The onset of petit mal in these
patients was about 2 years later than in patients with pure petit
mal. Patients with a simultaneous occurrence of petit mal and
grand mal revealed the latest onset of seizure at puberty.

5. In Chapter V correlations among paroxysmal EEG abnormalities
and other factors are analyzed. Paroxysmal EEG abnormalities,
especially sp-w-c, were frequently found in younger patients
and in those with a early onset of seizure. A decreased incidence
was noted with age. An increased frequency of patients with total
sp-w-c, atypical, 3.5-5/s, and with multiple sp-w-c was indicated
in female patients. In certain instances particular paroxysmal
EEG patterns correlated closely with certain types of seizures,
e.g., 3/s sp-w-c with absence PM and A-GM, temporal discharge
and psychomotor epilepsy. These correlations were determined by
coefficient contingency analyses. Some correlations between paroxysmal EEG abnormalities and basic EEG rhythm were observed.
Patients with sp-w-c (76 patients, 16 %) showed an increased incidence of patients with high voltage α-rhythm (20 %), β-waves
(20 %), slow waves (51 %), and with pathologic findings during
hyperventilation (84 %). On the other hand, no patient revealed
low voltage EEG (0 %) and only 3 patients (4 %) showed focal
sign in EEG. Patients with sp-w-c EEG abnormality were found to
show an increased frequency of familial predisposition to epilepsy (21 %), but a lower frequency in the presence of exogenous
factors (9 %).

6. Correlations between basic EEG rhythm and other factors were
analyzed. The number of patients with normal α-rhythm was less
at younger ages and in those with early onset. There were more
young patients with high voltage α-rhythm, among those with early
onset, in female patients, and in those with awakening GM, Lennox
syndrome, absence PM, myoclonic PM, paroxysmal and sp-w-c EEG,
and with familial predisposition to epilepsy. On the other hand,
the frequency was lower among those with S-GM, D-GM, and with
cortical epilepsy, and with slow waves in basic rhythm. Eighty-
one patients were observed with β-EEG (17 % of the total patients).
The incidence was increased in the age range of 10 - 39 years
(20 %), in those with age at onset of 5 - 19 years (22 %), in female patients (23 %), and in those with myoclonic PM (42 %) and
absence PM (21 %), total sp-w-c (20 %), and with familial predisposition to epilepsy (26 %). A decrease was observed after
the age of 40 years (8 %), and in those with S-GM (10 %).

One hundred and sixty-nine patients were observed with slow waves (36 % of the total patients). This abnormality was found more often at a younger age and in those with early onset, in those with A-GM (31 %), paroxysmal (82 %) and sp-w-c EEG (23 %), with pathologic changes during hyperventilation (37 %), and in those with exogenous factors (14 %); however, this abnormality was infrequent in patients with myoclonic PM and cortical epilepsy (7 %).

Thirteen patients were observed with low-voltage EEG (3 % of the total patients). These were all adults and non showed sp-w-c. This type of EEG increased in frequency in patients with occasional GM (62 %) and in those with cortical epilepsy (23 %), whereas it decreased in patients with A-GM (7 %), Lennox syndrome (0 %), and in those with absence PM (0 %).

One hundred and forty-two patients were observed with pathologic findings during hyperventilation (31 % of the total number). This abnormality was found more frequently among patients with A-GM (42 %), absence PM (51 %), and with myoclonic PM (60 %); whereas the frequency decreased in patients with S-GM (11 %), in D-GM (24 %), and in those with psychomotor epilepsy (20 %). Many of these patients showed typical (88 %) as well as atypical sp-w-c (83 %) and also familial predisposition to epilepsy (41 %).

Seventy-two patients were observed with focal sign in EEG (15 % of the total number). This abnormality was found with increased frequency among those with psychomotor (30 %) and cortical epilepsy (33 %). These patients also showed an increased frequency of the presence of exogenous factors (32 %). Focal sign was seldom found in patients with A-GM (7 %), absence PM (6 %), or in patients with sp-w-c (4 %).

In the present study, focal abnormality in EEG was found predominantly on the left side (71 %), and at the temporal area (75 %). The influence of the localization of focal abnormality, whether on the left or right side, temporal or other areas, was analyzed. Patients with left-sided focal EEG abnormality showed an earlier onset (0 - 9 years, 37 % vs. 24 % for patients with right-sided focal EEG abnormalities); a higher frequency of patients with grand mal during sleep (28 % vs. 5 %); an increased incidence of psychomotor epilepsy (53 % vs. 43 %) and of slow waves (47 % vs. 33 %); and a lower frequency of diffuse grand mal (16 % vs. 38 %), occasional grand mal (8 % vs. 33 %), and of total grand mal (63 % vs. 81 %), and the presence of exogenous factors (22 % vs. 38 %) than those with right-sided focal EEG abnormality.

Compared with those with extratemporal EEG abnormality, patients with temporal EEG abnormality were found to show a higher frequency in patients with grand mal during sleep (28 % vs. 0 %) and a higher incidence of psychomotor epilepsy (59 % vs. 22 %). A lower frequency in the presence of exogenous factors (17 % vs. 56 %) was observed in patients with temporal EEG abnormality.

7. Forty-six patients were identified with a familial predisposition to epilepsy (10 % of the total number). Familial predisposition occurred with an increased frequency in younger patients;

among those with earlier onset (0 - 9 years, 41 % vs. 26 % in those with no familial predisposition); and with an increased frequency in those with awakening grand mal (55 % vs. 31 %), absence PM (33 % vs. 13 %), and in those with sp-w-c (35 % vs. 14 %) as well as EEG abnormalities (59 % vs. 43 %). On the other hand, the frequency was lower in those with psychomotor epilepsy (17 % vs. 26 %) and the presence of exogenous factors (2 % vs. 14 %). Only one patient had both familial predisposition and exogenous factors.

8. Sixty patients were identified with exogenous factors (13 % of the total number). Patients with exogenous factors were predominantly male (80 % males and 20 % females). The number increased in patients aged 30 - 49 years, in those with age at onset of 0 - 1 and 20 - 39 years (48 %), in those with cortical epilepsy (22 %), in those with pathologic changes during hyperventilation (42 %), and in patients with focal sign in EEG (32 %). This was decreased in patients with teen-age onset (15 %), in those with awakening grand mal (18 %), with grand mal during sleep (10 %), and in patients with absence PM (3 %).

Appendix. Tables 1 – 45

Table 1. Distribution of patients by age and sex

Age (years)	Male n	%	Female n	%	Total n	%
5- 9	7	2.5	7	3.7	14	3.0
10-14	25	9.1	17	8.9	42	9.0
15-19	34	12.3	31	16.3	65	14.0
20-24	54	19.6	25	13.2	79	17.0
25-29	35	12.7	28	14.7	63	13.5
30-34	34	12.3	24	12.6	58	12.4
35-39	32	11.6	17	9.0	49	10.5
40-44	24	8.7	10	5.3	34	7.3
45-49	11	4.0	10	5.3	21	4.5
50-54	9	3.3	9	4.7	18	3.9
55-59	4	1.4	5	2.6	9	1.9
60-64	3	1.1	4	2.1	7	1.5
65-	4	1.4	3	1.6	7	1.5
Total	276	100.0	190	100.0	466	100.0

Table 2. Various findings in young, adult and aged patients

Age group	Total (N=466)		Young 5-19 years (N=121)			Adult 20-49 years (N=304)			Aged 50+ years (N=41)	
	n	%	n	%		n	%		n	%
Male patients	276	59.2	66	54.5		190	62.5		20	48.8
Female patients	190	40.8	55	45.5		114 ↓	37.5		21	51.2
Type of seizure										
Grand mal										
Awakening	147	31.5	43	35.5		97	31.9		7 ↓	17.1
Sleep	89	19.1	19	15.7		55	18.1	<	15 ↑	36.6
Diffuse	82	17.6	15	12.4		59	19.4		8	19.5
Occasional	76	16.3	23	19.0		48	15.8		5	12.2
Total	375	80.5	95	78.5		245	80.6		35	85.4
Petit mal										
Absence	70	15.0	27 ↑	22.3	>	40	13.2		3	7.3
Myoclonic	35	7.5	10	8.3 ⁻		25	8.2	>	0 ↓	-
Total	106	22.7	42 ↑	34.7	>	61	20.1		3 ↓	7.3
Psychomotor epilepsy	119	25.5	29	24.0		72	23.7	<	18 ↑	43.9
Cortical epilepsy	40	8.6	11	9.1		29	9.5	>	0 ↓	-
EEG										
Paroxysmal	276	59.2	89 ↑	73.6	>	164	53.9		23	56.1
Sp-w-c	76	16.3	33 ↑	27.3	>	40	13.2		3	7.3
Abnormal	208	44.6	67 ↑	55.4	>	127	41.8		14	34.1
High voltage α-wave	47	10.1	17	14.0		27	8.9		3	7.3
β-EEG	81	17.4	22	18.2		54	17.8		5	12.2
Slow waves	169	36.3	60 ↑	49.6	>	96	31.6		13	31.7
Low voltage EEG	13	2.8	0	-		13 ↑	4.3		0	-
Hyperventilation change	142	30.5	51 ↑	42.1	>	84	27.6		7	17.1
Focal sign	72	15.5	22	18.2		43	14.1		7	17.1
Familial predisposition	46	9.9	22 ↑	18.2	>	22	7.2		2	4.9
Exogenous factors	60	12.9	14	11.6		45	14.8	>	1 ↓	2.4

↑,↓ = statistically significantly increased or decreased when compared with
    other two age groups.

$\genfrac{}{}{0pt}{}{>}{<}$ = statistically significant difference between two age groups.

Table 3. Distribution of patients by age at onset of seizure

Age at onset of seizure (years)	Male		Female		Total	
	n	%	n	%	n	%
0- 1	14	5.1	6	3.2	20	4.3
2- 4	15	5.4	15	7.9	30	6.4
5- 9	38	13.8	42	22.1	80	17.2
10-14	58	21.0	42	22.1	100	21.4
15-19	39	14.1	24	12.7	63	13.5
20-24	34	12.3	16	8.4	50	10.7
25-29	20	7.3	16	8.4	36	7.7
30-34	23	8.3	9	4.7	32	6.9
35-39	10	3.6	9	4.7	19	4.1
40-44	11	4.0	3	1.6	14	3.0
45-49	8	2.9	3	1.6	11	2.4
50-54	1	0.4	1	0.5	2	0.4
55-59	3	1.1	1	0.5	4	0.9
60-	2	0.7	3	1.6	5	1.1
Total	276	100.0	190	100.0	466	100.0

Table 4. Distribution of patients by types of seizures[a]

Type of seizure	Male		Female		Total	
	n	%	n	%	n	%
Grand mal						
Awakening	84	30.4	63	33.2	147	31.5
Sleep	53	19.2	36	18.9	89	19.1
Diffuse	50	18.1	32	16.8	82	17.6
Occasional	45	16.3	31	16.3	76	16.3
Total	221	80.1	154	81.1	375	80.5
Petit mal						
West	2	0.7	1	0.5	3	0.6
Lennox	2	0.7	3	1.6	5	1.1
Absence	35	12.7	35	18.4	70	15.0
Myoclonic	19	6.9	16	8.4	35	7.5
Total	54	19.6	52	27.4	106	22.7
Psychomotor epilepsy	65	23.5	54	28.7	119	25.5
Cortical eplilepsy	29	10.5	11	5.8	40	8.6
Total	276		190		466	

[a]Some patients had more than one type of seizure.

Table 5. Distribution of patients by pure type of seizure

Pure type of seizure	Male			Female			Total			n/N
	N	n	%	N	n	%	N	n	%	
Grand mal										
Awakening	84	33	22.1	63	20	24.7	147	53	23.0	36.0
Sleep	53	27	18.1	36	12	14.8	89	39	17.0	43.8
Diffuse	50	21	14.1	32	10	12.3	82	31	13.5	37.8
Occasional	45	32	21.5	31	17	21.0	76	49	21.3	64.5
Total	221	113	75.8	154	59	72.8	375	172	74.8	45.9
Petit mal										
West	2	0	–	1	1	1.2	3	1	0.4	33.3
Lennox	2	1	0.7	3	0	–	5	1	0.4	20.0
Absence	35	5	3.3	35	4	4.9	70	9	3.9	12.8
Myoclonic	19	2	1.3	16	3	3.7	35	5	2.2	14.3
Total	54	8	5.4	52	8	9.9	106	16	7.0	15.0
Psychomotor epilepsy	65	15	10.1	54	9	11.1	119	24	10.4	20.2
Cortical epilepsy	29	13	8.7	11	5	6.2	40	18	7.8	45.0
Total	276	149	100.0	190	81	100.0	466	230	100.0	49.4
n/N %		(54.0)			(42.6)			(49.4)		

N: Total number of patients with certain types of seizures.

n: Number of patients with pure type of seizures.

Table 6. Distribution of patients by types of paroxysmal EEG patterns

Paroxysmal EEG patterns	Male		Female		Total	
	n	%	n	%	n	%
Number of patients with paroxysmal EEG abnormalities	157	56.9	119	62.6	276	59.2
Spike-wave-complex						
3/s sp-w-c	12	4.3	12	6.3	24	5.1
Atypical sp-w-c	22	8.O	3O	15.8	52	11.2
Total sp-w-c	34	12.3	42	22.1	76	16.3
Sharp and slow waves	24	8.7	13	6.8	37	7.9
Spikes	7	2.5	1	O.5	8	1.7
Sharp waves	84	30.4	54	28.4	138	29.6
Temporal discharge	8	2.9	9	4.7	17	3.6
Total	276		190		466	

Table 7. Distribution of patients by basic EEG rhythm and EEG diagnosis

EEG	Male		Female		Total	
	n	%	n	%	n	%
α-waves						
Normal α	232	84.1	136	71.6	368	78.9
High voltage α	19	6.9	28	14.7	47	10.1
No α	25	9.1	26	13.7	51	10.9
β-EEG	38	13.8	43	22.6	81	17.4
Slow waves	98	35.5	71	37.4	169	36.3
θ-wave	52	18.8	42	22.1	94	20.2
θ-δ-waves	46	16.7	29	15.3	75	16.1
Low voltage EEG	9	3.3	4	2.1	13	2.8
Hyperventilation						
Pathologic change	83	30.1	59	31.1	142	30.5
Focal sign	44	15.9	28	14.7	72	15.4
EEG diagnosis						
Normal	75	27.2	40	21.1	115	24.7
Borderline	83	30.1	60	31.6	143	30.7
Abnormal	41	14.8	23	12.1	64	13.7
Epileptic	37	13.4	43	22.6	80	17.2
Focal	40	14.5	24	12.6	64	13.7
Total	276		190		466	

Table 8. Distribution of patients by familial predisposition and exogenous factors

	Male		Female		Total	
	n	%	n	%	n	%
Familial disposition	30	10.9	16	8.4	46	9.9
Exogenous factors	48	17.4	12	6.3	60	12.9

Table 9. Correlation between types of seizures and age (males)

Age	Grand mal										Petit			
(years)	A		S		D		O		Total		West		Lennox	
	n	%	n	%	n	%	n	%	n	%	n	%	n	%
5- 9	2	2.4	0	-	0	-	2	4.4	4	1.8	0	-	0	-
10-14	6	7.1	3	5.7	5	10.0	5	11.1	18	8.1	1	50.0	1	50.0
15-19	13	15.5	7	13.2	6	12.0	5	11.1	31	14.0	1	50.0	1	50.0
20-24	24	28.6	9	17.0	6	12.0	8	17.8	46	20.8	0	-	0	-
25-29	8	9.5	6	11.3	10	20.0	5	11.1	26	11.8	0	-	0	-
30-34	11	13.1	4	7.5	4	8.0	9	20.0	28	12.7	0	-	0	-
35-39	8	9.5	9	17.0	6	12.0	5	11.1	25	11.3	0	-	0	-
40-44	4	4.8	6	11.3	6	12.0	5	11.1	18	8.1	0	-	0	-
45-49	3	3.6	2	3.8	3	6.0	0	-	8	3.6	0	-	0	-
50-54	3	3.6	2	3.8	2	4.0	1	2.2	8	3.6	0	-	0	-
55-59	1	1.2	2	3.8	1	2.0	0	-	4	1.8	0	-	0	-
60-64	0	-	1	1.9	1	2.0	0	-	2	0.9	0	-	0	-
65-	1	1.2	2	3.8	0	-	0	-	3	1.4	0	-	0	-
Total	84	30.4	53	19.2	50	18.1	45	16.3	221	80.1	2	0.7	2	0.7

Table 10. Correlation between types of seizures and age (females)

Age	Grand mal										Petit			
(years)	A		S		D		O		Total		West		Lennox	
	n	%	n	%	n	%	n	%	n	%	n	%	n	%
5- 9	0	-	2	5.6	0	-	2	6.5	4	2.6	0	-	0	-
10-14	6	9.5	2	5.6	0	-	4	12.9	12	7.8	0	-	1	33.3
15-19	16	25.4	5	13.9	4	12.5	5	16.1	16	10.4	1	100.0	2	66.7
20-24	7	11.1	6	16.7	4	12.5	4	12.9	19	12.3	0	-	0	-
25-29	11	17.5	3	8.3	4	12.5	2	6.5	19	12.3	0	-	0	-
30-34	8	12.7	1	2.8	8	25.0	6	19.4	23	14.9	0	-	0	-
35-39	7	11.1	3	8.3	4	12.5	2	6.5	15	9.7	0	-	0	-
40-44	4	6.3	2	5.6	2	6.3	1	3.2	9	5.8	0	-	0	-
45-49	2	3.2	4	11.1	2	6.3	1	3.2	9	5.8	0	-	0	-
50-54	1	1.6	3	8.3	0	-	3	9.7	7	4.5	0	-	0	-
55-59	1	1.6	3	8.3	1	3.1	0	-	5	3.2	0	-	0	-
60-64	0	-	1	2.8	2	6.3	0	-	3	1.9	0	-	0	-
65-	0	-	1	2.8	1	3.1	1	3.2	3	1.9	0	-	0	-
Total	63	33.2	36	18.9	32	16.8	31	16.3	154	81.1	1	0.5	3	1.5

mal						Psychomotor epilepsy		Cortical epilepsy		Total number of patients	
Absence		Myoclonic		Total							
n	%	n	%	n	%	n	%	n	%	n	%
3	8.6	0	–	3	5.6	1	1.5	2	6.9	7	2.5
4	11.4	2	10.5	8	14.8	7	10.8	3	10.3	25	9.1
7	20.2	3	15.8	10	18.5	4	6.2	3	10.3	34	12.3
11	31.4	6	31.6	16	29.6	11	16.9	8	27.6	54	19.6
1	2.9	4	21.5	5	9.3	9	13.8	2	6.9	35	12.7
4	11.4	1	5.3	5	9.3	8	12.3	4	13.8	34	12.3
2	5.7	3	15.8	4	7.4	9	13.8	4	13.8	32	11.6
2	5.7	0	–	2	3.7	5	7.7	2	6.9	24	8.7
1	2.9	0	–	1	1.9	2	3.1	0	–	11	4.0
0	–	0	–	0	–	4	6.2	0	–	9	3.3
0	–	0	–	0	–	1	1.5	0	–	4	1.4
0	–	0	–	0	–	2	3.1	0	–	3	1.1
0	–	0	–	0	–	2.	3.1	0	–	4	1.4
35	12.7	19	6.9	54	19.6	65	23.6	29	10.5	276	100.0

mal						Psychomotor epilepsy		Cortical epilepsy		Total number of patients	
Absence		Myoclonic		Total							
n	%	n	%	n	%	n	%	n	%	n	%
2	5.7	0	–	2	3.8	0	–	0	–	7	3.7
5	14.3	0		6	11.5	8	14.8	2	18.2	17	9.0
6	17.1	5	31.2	13	25.0	9	16.7	1	9.1	31	16.3
6	17.1	2	12.5	7	13.5	6	11.1	2	18.2	25	13.2
3	8.6	4	25.0	6	11.5	7	13.0	1	9.1	28	14.7
2	5.7	4	25.0	6	11.5	4	7.4	3	27.3	24	12.6
4	11.4	1	6.3	5	9.6	4	7.4	1	9.1	17	8.9
3	8.6	0	–	3	5.8	4	7.4	0	–	10	5.3
1	2.9	0	–	1	1.9	3	5.6	1	9.1	10	5.3
1	2.9	0	–	1	1.9	3	5.6	0	–	9	4.7
1	2.9	0	–	1	1.9	3	5.6	0	–	5	2.6
1	2.9	0	–	1	1.9	2	3.7	0	–	4	2.1
0	–	0	–	0	–	1	1.9	0	–	3	1.6
35	18.4	16	8.4	52	27.4	54	28.4	11	5.8	190	100.0

Table 11. Types of seizures and the age at onset (males)

Age at onset (years)	Number of patients	Grand mal									
		A		S		D		O		Total	
		n	%	n	%	n	%	n	%	n	%
0- 1	14	3	3.6	1	1.9	7	14.0	1	2.2	11	5.0
2- 4	15	4	4.8	1	1.9	4	8.0	1	2.2	10	4.5
5- 9	38	16	19.0	7	13.2	4	8.0	4	8.9	29	13.1
10-14	58	18	21.4	14	26.4	9	18.0	13	28.9	52	23.5
15-19	39	17	20.2	8	15.1	6	12.0	3	6.7	33	14.9
20-24	34	12	14.3	7	13.2	4	8.0	7	15.6	29	13.1
25-29	20	2	2.4	2	3.8	7	14.0	5	11.1	15	6.8
30-34	23	7	8.3	4	7.5	4	8.0	4	8.9	17	7.7
35-39	10	0	-	2	3.8	2	4.0	4	8.9	7	3.2
40-44	11	1	1.2	2	3.8	2	4.0	3	6.7	8	3.6
45-49	8	4	4.8	1	1.9	1	2.0	0	-	6	2.7
50-	6	0	-	4	7.5	0	-	0	-	4	1.8
Total	276	84		53		50		45		221	

Table 12. Types of seizures and the age at onset (females)

Age at onset (years)	Number of patients	Grand mal									
		A		S		D		O		Total	
		n	%	n	%	n	%	n	%	n	%
0- 1	6	1	1.6	1	2.8	1	3.1	1	3.2	4	2.6
2- 4	15	3	4.8	3	8.3	3	9.4	3	9.7	12	7.8
5- 9	42	16	25.4	5	13.9	8	25.0	7	22.6	34	22.1
10-14	42	22	34.9	9	25.0	5	15.6	4	12.9	36	23.4
15-19	24	13	20.6	1	2.8	2	6.3	2	6.5	18	11.7
20-24	16	4	6.3	4	11.1	6	18.8	2	6.5	15	9.7
25-29	16	2	3.2	1	2.8	3	9.4	5	16.1	11	7.1
30-34	9	2	3.2	1	2.8	2	6.3	2	6.5	6	3.9
35-39	9	0	-	4	11.1	0	-	3	9.7	7	4.5
40-44	3	0	-	3	8.3	0	-	0	-	3	1.9
45-49	3	0	-	3	8.3	0	-	0	-	3	1.9
50-	5	0	-	1	2.8	2	6.3	2	6.5	5	3.2
Total	190	63		36		32		31		154	

Petit mal										Psychomotor epilepsy		Cortical epilepsy	
West		Lennox		Absence		Myoclonic		Total					
n	%	n	%	n	%	n	%	n	%	n	%	n	%
1	50.0	1	50.0	0	-	0	-	2	3.7	9	13.8	1	3.4
1	50.0	1	50.0	5	14.3	0	-	7	13.0	3	4.6	1	3.4
0	-	0	-	13	37.1	2	10.5	14	25.9	7	10.8	8	27.6
0	-	0	-	11	31.4	8	42.1	16	29.6	9	13.8	4	13.8
0	-	0	-	4	11.4	5	26.3	9	16.7	5	7.7	6	20.7
0	-	0	-	0	-	4	21.1	4	7.4	12	18.5	3	10.3
0	-	0	-	1	2.9	0	-	1	1.9	7	10.8	1	3.4
0	-	0	-	1	2.9	0	-	1	1.9	4	6.2	2	6.9
0	-	0	-	0	-	0	-	0	-	2	3.1	1	3.4
0	-	0	-	0	-	0	-	0	-	2	3.1	1	3.4
0	-	0	-	0	-	0	-	0	-	1	1.5	1	3.4
0	-	0	-	0	-	0	-	0	-	4	6.2	0	-
2		2		35		19		54		65		29	

Petit mal										Psychomotor epilepsy		Cortical epilepsy	
West		Lennox		Absence		Myoclonic		Total					
n	%	n	%	n	%	n	%	n	%	n	%	n	%
1	100.0	1	33.3	0	-	0	-	2	3.8	3	5.6	1	9.1
0	-	1	33.3	1	2.9	2	12.5	3	5.8	5	9.3	1	9.1
0	-	1	33.3	23	65.7	3	18.8	26	50.0	9	16.7	2	18.1
0	-	0	-	8	22.9	6	37.5	13	25.0	12	22.2	1	9.1
0	-	0	-	1	2.9	5	31.3	6	11.5	4	7.4	3	27.3
0	-	0	-	0	-	0	-	0	-	7	13.0	0	-
0	-	0	-	2	5.7	0	-	2	3.8	4	7.4	1	9.1
0	-	0	-	0	-	0	-	0	-	2	3.7	1	9.1
0	-	0	-	0	-	0	-	0	-	3	5.6	1	9.1
0	-	0	-	0	-	0	-	0	-	2	3.7	0	-
0	-	0	-	0	-	0	-	0	-	2	3.7	0	-
0	-	0	-	0	-	0	-	0	-	1	1.9	0	-
1		3		35		16		52		54		11	

Table 13. Peak or age range at onset in different types of seizures

Type of seizure	Peak or age range at onset (years)	Reference
Grand mal		
Awakening	16	JANZ (1955)
	6-15	FURUICHI (1969)
	(6)8-15 (22)[a]	
Sleep	No peak in children	KRUSE (1964)
	nor in adults	JANZ (1955)
	6-10	FURUICHI (1969)
	35+[a]	
Diffuse	0 - 5 and 11-15	FURUICHI (1969)
	0-4[a]	
Petit mal		
West syndrome	3- 6 - 9 months	LENNOX and DAVIS (1950)
		KELLAWAY (1952)
Lennox syndrome	2- 3 - 4	DOOSE (1964b, c)
	1- 4[a]	
Absence	4- 6- 7 - 8	LENNOX and DAVIS (1950)
		O'BRIEN et al. (1959)
		CURRIER et al. (1963)
	5-12[a]	
Myoclonic	14-18 (20)	JANZ and CHRISTIAN (1957)
	10-19	DALBY (1969)
	10-15 (20)[a]	
Psychomotor epilepsy	0- 4	LENNOX and DAVIS (1950)
	1-15	GIBBS and GIBBS (1952)
	No peak in adults	JANZ (1969)
	0-5 and 20-29[a]	
Cortical epilepsy	5-19[a]	

[a] Present study.

Table 14. Correlation between types of seizure and paroxysmal EEG patterns

Paroxysmal EEG patterns	Grand mal									
	A		S		D		O		Total	
	n	%	n	%	n	%	n	%	n	%
1. Sp-w-c										
3/s sp-w-c	9	10.7	0	–	1	2.0	1	2.2	11	5.0
Atypical sp-w-c	14	16.7	1	1.9	2	4.0	2	4.4	19	8.6
Total sp-w-c	23	27.4	1	1.9	3	6.0	3	6.6	30	13.6
2. Sharp and slow waves	11	13.1	5	9.4	5	10.0	3	6.7	21	9.5
3. Spikes	2	2.4	1	1.9	1	2.0	1	2.2	5	2.3
4. Sharp waves	23	27.4	13	24.5	20	40.0	14	31.1	65	29.4
5. Temporal discharge	1	1.2	2	3.8	2	4.0	1	2.2	6	2.7
Number of patients with paroxysmal patterns	60	71.4	22	41.5	31	62.0	22	48.9	127	57.5
Total number of patients	84		53		50		45		221	

Table 15. Correlation between types of seizures and paroxysmal EEG patterns

Paroxysmal EEG patterns	Grand mal									
	A		S		D		O		Total	
	n	%	n	%	n	%	n	%	n	%
1. Sp-w-c										
3/s sp-w-c	10	15.9	0	–	1	3.1	2	6.5	12	7.8
Atypical sp-w-c	16	25.4	0	–	2	6.3	6	19.4	24	15.6
Total sp-w-c	26	41.3	0	–	3	9.4	8	25.8	36	23.4
2. Sharp and slow waves	2	3.2	2	5.6	2	6.3	2	6.5	8	5.2
3. Spikes	1	1.6	0	–	0	–	0	–	1	0.6
4. Sharp waves	13	20.6	15	41.7	7	21.9	7	22.6	40	26.0
5. Temporal discharge	3	4.8	2	5.6	0	–	1	3.2	6	3.9
Number of patients with paroxysmal patterns	45	71.4	19	52.8	12	37.5	18	58.1	96	62.3
Total	63		36		32		31		154	

(males)

Petit mal										Psycho-motor epilepsy		Cortical epilepsy		Total number of patients	
West		Lennox		Absence		Myoclonic		Total							
n	%	n	%	n	%	n	%	n	%	n	%	n	%	n	%
O	–	O	–	7	20.0	4	21.1	9	16.7	1	1.5	1	3.4	12	4.3
2	100.0	1	50.0	7	20.0	5	26.3	14	25.9	O	–	O	–	22	8.0
2	100.0	1	50.0	14	40.0	9	47.4	23	42.6	1	1.5	1	3.4	34	12.3
O	–	O	–	1	2.9	4	21.1	4	7.4	5	7.7	3	10.3	24	8.7
O	–	O	–	1	2.9	O	–	1	1.9	3	4.6	1	3.4	7	2.5
O	–	1	50.0	9	25.7	3	15.8	13	24.1	27	41.5	9	31.0	84	30.4
O	–	O	–	1	2.9	O	–	1	1.9	6	9.2	1	3.4	8	2.9
2	100.0	2	100.0	26	74.3	16	84.2	42	77.8	42	64.6	15	51.7	157	56.9
2		2		35		19		54		65		29		276	

(females)

Petit mal										Psycho-motor epilepsy		Cortical epilepsy		Total number of patients	
West		Lennox		Absence		Myoclonic		Total							
n	%	n	%	n	%	n	%	n	%	n	%	n	%	n	%
O	–	O	–	6	17.1	2	12.5	8	15.4	1	1.9	O	–	12	6.3
O	–	2	100.0	6	17.1	6	37.5	13	25.0	7	13.0	2	18.2	30	15.8
O	–	2	100.0	12	34.3	8	50.0	21	40.4	8	14.8	2	18.2	42	22.1
O	–	O	–	3	8.6	O	–	3	5.8	6	11.1	1	9.1	13	6.8
O	–	O	–	O	–	O	–	O	–	O	–	O	–	1	0.5
O	50.0	1	50.0	9	25.7	5	31.3	15	28.8	17	31.5	5	45.5	54	28.4
O	–	O	–	1	2.9	O	–	1	1.9	6	11.1	1	9.1	9	4.7
O	–	3	100.0	25	71.4	13	81.3	40	76.9	37	68.5	9	81.8	119	62.6
1		3		35		16		52		54		11		190	

Table 16. Relative coefficient of contingency on the correlation between

Type of seizure	Sp-w-c			Temporal discharge	Total paroxysmal
	3/s	atypical	total		
Grand mal					
Awakening	.604	.427	.447	-.394	.341
Sleep	-1.000	-.896	-.931	.154	-.257
Diffuse	.463	-.542	-.578	.003	-.131
Occasional	-.118	-.058	-.119	-.028	-.127
Petit mal					
Lennox	.000	.505	.465	-1.000	1.000
Absence	.520	.154	.336	-.079	.357
Myoclonic	.245	.291	.401	-1.000	.605
Psychomotor epilepsy	-.838	-.498	-.562	.614	.196
Cortical epilepsy	-.361	-.489	-.504	.066	.020

Figures in the 5 columns on the right side include each paroxysmal potential.

Table 17. Correlation between types of seizure and paroxysmal EEG patterns in

Paroxysmal EEG patterns	Grand mal									
	A		S		D		O		Total	
	n	%	n	%	n	%	n	%	n	%
Sp-w-c										
3/s sp-w-c	9	10.7	0	–	1	2.0	1	2.2	11	5.0
irregular sp-w-c	8	9.5	0	–	1	2.0	0	–	9	4.1
2-2.5/s sp-w-c	4	4.8	0	–	2	4.0	0	–	6	2.7
3.5-5/s sp-w-c	3	3.6	1	1.9	1	2.0	1	2.2	6	2.7
Multiple sp-w-c	10	11.9	0	–	2	4.0	1	2.2	13	5.9
Sharp and slow waves	14	16.7	6	11.3	5	10.0	4	8.9	29	13.1
Spikes	8	9.5	1	1.9	1	2.0	2	4.4	12	5.4
Sharp waves	42	50.0	17	32.1	23	46.0	18	40.0	100	45.2
Temporal discharge	2	2.4	4	7.5	4	8.0	3	6.7	13	5.9
Number of patients with paroxysmal patterns	60	71.4	22	41.5	31	62.0	22	48.9	127	57.5
Total number of patients	84		53		50		45		221	
Total number of scores	100		29		40		30		199	

types of seizure and paroxysmal EEG abnormalities

	Sp-w-c			Sharp waves
irregular	2-2.5/s	3.5-5/s	multiple	
.476	.535	.385	.643	.056
-1.000	-1.000	-.768	-1.000	-.196
.325	.000	-.745	-.247	-.088
-.317	-.099	.000	-.695	-.074
.032	.076	.286	.000	.013
.246	.351	.189	.341	.104
.104	.005	.038	.161	.341
-.178	-.051	-.832	-.749	.124
-.231	.000	-.392	-.496	.072

male patients (each paroxysmal pattern was registered)

Petit mal										Psycho-motor epilepsy		Cortical epilepsy		Total number of	
West		Lennox		Absence		Myoclonic		Total						scores	pa-tients
n	%	n	%	n	%	n	%	n	%	n	%	n	%		
O	-	O	-	7	20.0	4	21.1	11	20.4	1	1.5	1	3.4	24	12
1	50.0	O	-	5	14.3	4	21.1	10	18.5	O	-	O	-	19	11
O		O	-	3	8.6	1	5.3	4	7.4	O	-	O	-	10	6
O	-	O	-	4	11.4	O	-	4	7.4	O	-	O	-	10	7
1	50.0	1	50.0	5	14.3	3	15.8	10	18.5	O	-	1	3.4	24	14
O	-	O	-	5	14.3	5	26.3	10	18.5	5	7.7	3	10.3	47	28
O	-	1	50.0	2	5.7	1	5.3	4	7.4	3	4.6	1	3.4	20	15
2	100.0	2	100.0	17	48.6	9	47.4	30	55.6	32	49.2	13	44.8	175	120
O	-	O	-	2	5.7	O	-	2	3.7	10	15.4	2	6.9	27	14
2	100.0	2	100.0	26	74.3	16	84.2	42	77.8	42	64.6	15	51.7	226	157
2		2		35		19		54		65		29		-	276
4		4		50		27		85		51		21		356	-

Table 18. Correlation between types of seizure and paroxysmal EEG patterns in

Paroxysmal EEG patterns	Grand mal									
	A		S		D		O		Total	
	n	%	n	%	n	%	n	%	n	%
Sp-w-c										
3/s sp-w-c	10	15.9	0	–	1	3.1	2	6.5	13	8.4
irregular sp-w-c	5	7.9	0	–	1	3.1	2	6.5	8	5.2
2-2.5/s sp-w-c	3	4.8	0	–	0	–	1	3.2	4	2.6
3.5-5/s sp-w-c	11	17.5	0	–	0	–	3	9.7	14	9.1
Multiple sp-w-c	14	22.2	0	–	2	6.3	1	3.2	17	11.0
Sharp and slow waves	4	6.3	2	5.6	3	9.4	3	9.7	12	7.8
Spikes	4	6.3	1	2.8	0	–	1	3.2	6	3.9
Sharp waves	26	41.3	15	41.7	10	31.3	13	41.9	64	41.6
Temporal discharge	3	4.8	2	5.6	1	3.1	1	3.2	7	4.5
Number of patients with paroxysmal patterns	45	71.4	19	52.8	12	37.5	18	58.1	91	59.1
Total number of patients	63		36		32		31		154	
Total number of scores	80		20		18		27		145	

female patients (each paroxysmal pattern was registered)

West		Lennox		Absence		Myoclonic		Total		Psycho-motor epilepsy		Cortical epilepsy		Total number of	
n	%	n	%	n	%	n	%	n	%	n	%	n	%	scores	patients
O	–	O	–	6	17.1	2	12.5	8	15.4	1	1.9	O	–	22	12
O	–	O	–	2	5.7	1	6.3	3	5.8	4	7.4	1	9.1	16	10
O	–	1	50.0	1	2.9	1	6.3	3	5.8	1	1.9	1	9.1	9	5
O	–	1	50.0	4	11.4	4	25.0	9	17.3	1	1.9	1	9.1	25	18
O	–	O	–	8	22.9	3	18.8	11	21.2	2	3.7	O	–	30	19
O	–	O	–	4	11.4	O	–	4	7.7	6	11.1	1	9.1	23	17
O	–	O	–	2	5.7	2	12.5	4	7.7	2	3.7	O	–	12	10
2	66.7	O	–	16	45.7	9	56.3	27	51.9	27	50.0	6	54.5	124	85
1	33.3	O	–	1	2.9	O	–	2	3.8	7	13.0	1	9.1	17	11
2	66.7	1	100.0	25	71.4	13	81.3	40	76.9	37	68.5	9	81.8	177	119
3		1		35		16		52		54		11		–	190
3		2		44		22		71		51		11		278	

Table 19. Correlation between types of seizure and EEG, focal sign, pathologic exogenous factors (males)

	Grand mal									
	A		S		D		O		Total	
	n	%	n	%	n	%	n	%	n	%
α-EEG										
Normal α	68	81.0	45	84.9	43	86.0	37	82.2	185	83.7
High voltage α	9	10.7	0	–	3	6.0	3	6.7	15	6.8
Without α	7	8.3	8	15.1	4	8.0	5	11.1	21	9.5
β-EEG	13	15.5	4	7.5	4	8.0	6	13.3	26	11.8
θ- and δ-waves	27	32.1	24	45.3	19	38.0	14	31.1	80	36.2
θ-wave	16	19.0	11	20.0	11	22.0	6	13.3	44	19.9
θ-δ-waves	11	13.1	13	24.5	8	16.0	8	17.8	36	16.3
Low voltage EEG	1	1.2	1	1.9	1	2.0	5	11.1	8	3.6
Focal sign	6	7.1	7	13.2	11	22.0	9	22.0	30	13.6
Hyperventilation pathologic change	35	41.7	7	13.2	14	28.0	11	24.4	65	29.4
EEG diagnosis										
a) normal	20	23.8	18	34.0	14	28.0	14	31.1	62	28.0
b) borderline	19	22.6	17	32.1	17	34.0	15	33.3	66	29.9
c) abnormal	17	20.2	8	15.1	6	12.0	3	6.7	33	14.9
d) epileptic	23	27.4	3	5.7	3	6.0	5	11.1	33	14.9
e) focal	5	6.0	7	13.2	10	20.0	8	17.8	27	12.2
c),d),e)	45	53.6	18	34.0	19	38.0	16	35.6	93	42.1
Familial predisposition	11	13.1	5	9.4	6	12.0	3	6.7	25	11.3
Exogenous factors	7	8.3	5	9.4	12	24.0	11	24.4	33	14.9
Total number of patients	84		53		50		45		221	

change during hyperventilation, EEG diagnosis, familial predisposition, and

West		Lennox		Petit mal						Psycho-motor epilepsy		Cortical epilepsy		Total number of patients	
				Absence		Myoclonic		Total							
n	%	n	%	n	%	n	%	n	%	n	%	n	%	n	%
1	50.0	O	-	31	88.6	14	73.7	43	79.6	53	81.5	27	93.1	232	84.1
O	-	O	-	3	8.6	3	15.8	6	11.1	5	7.7	O	-	19	6.9
1	50.0	2	100.0	1	2.9	2	10.5	5	9.3	7	10.8	2	6.9	25	9.1
O	-	O	-	4	11.4	6	31.6	10	18.5	8	12.3	6	20.7	38	13.8
1	50.0	2	100.0	15	42.9	5	26.3	22	40.7	28	43.1	7	24.1	98	35.5
2	100.0	1	50.0	7	20.0	3	15.8	12	22.2	14	21.5	3	10.3	52	18.8
O	-	1	50.0	8	22.9	2	10.5	10	18.5	14	21.5	4	13.8	46	16.7
O	-	O	-	O	-	O	-	1	1.9	2	3.1	3	10.3	9	3.3
O	-	1	50.0	3	8.6	2	10.5	6	11.1	20	30.8	9	31.0	44	15.9
O	-	O	-	19	54.3	12	63.2	29	53.7	14	21.5	8	27.6	83	30.1
O	-	O	-	6	17.1	1	5.3	7	13.0	10	15.4	6	20.7	75	27.2
O	-	O	-	9	25.7	4	21.1	12	22.2	19	29.2	10	34.5	83	30.1
O	-	O	-	5	14.3	3	15.8	8	14.8	15	23.1	2	6.9	41	14.9
2	100.0	1	50.0	13	37.1	9	47.4	22	40.7	1	1.5	2	6.9	37	13.4
O	-	1	50.0	2	5.7	2	10.5	5	9.3	20	30.8	9	31.0	40	14.5
2	100.0	2	100.0	20	57.1	14	73.1	35	64.8	36	55.4	13	44.8	118	42.8
O	-	O	-	9	25.7	3	15.8	11	20.4	3	4.6	3	10.3	30	10.9
1	50.0	O	-	1	2.9	3	15.8	5	9.3	9	13.8	10	34.5	48	17.4
2		2		35		19		54		65		29		276	

Table 20. Correlation between types of seizures and EEG, focal sign, pathologic exogenous factors (females)

	Grand mal									
	A		S		D		O		Total	
	n	%	n	%	n	%	n	%	n	%
α-EEG										
Normal α	43	68.3	29	80.6	25	78.1	21	67.7	112	72.7
High voltage α	12	19.0	4	11.1	4	12.5	3	9.7	22	14.3
Without α	8	12.7	3	8.3	3	9.4	7	22.6	20	13.0
β-EEG	17	27.0	5	13.9	6	18.8	6	19.4	31	20.1
θ- and δ-waves	25	39.7	11	30.6	10	31.3	15	48.4	58	37.7
θ-wave	13	20.6	6	16.7	8	25.0	11	35.5	36	23.4
θ-δ-waves	12	19.0	5	13.9	2	6.3	4	12.9	22	14.3
Low voltage EEG	0	–	1	2.8	0	–	3	9.7	4	2.6
Focal sign	4	6.3	8	22.2	5	15.6	2	6.5	19	12.3
Hyperventilation pathologic change	27	42.9	3	8.3	6	18.8	11	35.5	46	29.9
EEG diagnosis										
a) normal	15	23.8	9	25.0	10	31.3	6	19.4	38	24.7
b) borderline	14	22.2	13	36.1	12	37.5	13	41.9	48	31.2
c) abnormal	5	7.9	6	16.7	3	9.4	3	9.7	16	10.4
d) epileptic	26	41.3	1	2.8	2	6.3	8	25.8	36	23.4
e) focal	3	4.8	7	19.4	5	15.6	1	3.2	16	10.4
c),d),e)	34	54.0	14	38.9	10	31.3	12	38.7	68	44.2
Familial predisposition	5	7.9	1	2.8	0	–	3	9.7	9	5.8
Exogenous factors	4	6.3	1	2.8	1	3.1	3	9.7	9	5.8
Total number of patients	63		36		32		31		154	

change during hyperventilation, EEG diagnosis, familial predisposition, and

				Petit mal								Psycho-motor epilepsy		Cortical epilepsy		Total number of patients	
West		Lennox		Absence		Myoclonic		Total									
n	%	n	%	n	&	n	%	n	%			n	%	n	%	n	%
1	100.0	1	33.3	23	65.7	13	81.3	35	67.3			36	66.7	9	81.8	136	71.6
O	-	O	-	6	17.1	2	12.5	8	15.4			8	14.8	O	-	28	14.7
O	-	2	66.7	6	17.1	1	6.3	9	17.3			10	18.5	2	18.2	26	13.7
O	-	1	33.3	11	31.4	8	50.0	18	34.6			14	25.9	4	36.4	43	22.6
1	100.0	2	66.7	13	37.1	3	18.8	19	36.5			17	31.5	4	36.4	71	37.4
1	100.0	O	-	8	22.9	1	6.3	10	19.2			12	22.2	2	18.2	42	22.1
O	-	2	66.7	5	14.3	2	12.5	9	17.3			5	9.3	2	18.2	29	15.3
O	-	O	-	O	-	O	-	O	-			1	1.9	O	-	4	2.1
O	-	1	33.3	1	2.9	O	-	2	3.8			16	29.6	4	36.4	28	14.7
O	-	1	33.3	17	48.6	9	56.3	26	50.0			10	18.5	4	36.4	59	31.1
1	100.0	O	-	8	22.9	2	12.5	9	17.3			7	13.0	1	9.1	40	21.1
O	-	O	-	9	25.7	5	31.3	14	26.9			19	35.2	2	18.2	60	31.6
O	-	O	-	3	8.6	1	6.3	4	7.7			10	18.5	2	18.2	23	12.1
O	-	2	66.7	14	40.0	8	50.0	23	44.2			6	11.1	2	18.2	43	22.6
O	-	1	33.3	1	2.9	O	-	1	1.9			12	22.2	4	36.4	24	12.6
O	-	2	66.7	18	51.4	9	56.3	29	55.8			28	51.9	8	72.7	90	47.4
O	-	1	33.3	6	17.1	1	6.3	8	15.4			5	9.3	1	9.1	16	8.4
O	-	O	-	1	2.9	1	6.3	2	3.8			2	3.7	3	27.3	12	6.3
1		3		35		16		52				54		11		190	

Table 21. Types of seizure and incidence of familial predisposition

Type of seizure	Minimum and reference	Median	Maximum and reference
Petit mal			
West syndrome	7% GIBBS et al. (1954)	17%	25% BAMBERGER and MATTHES (1959)
Lennox syndrome	16% KRUSE (1968)	32%	42% BUENO et al. (1970)
Absence PM	10% HERTOFT (1963)	19%	44% CURRIER et al. (1963)
Myoclonic PM	17% JANZ and CHRISTIAN (1957)	23%	37% CASTELLS and MENDILAHARSU (1958)
Grand mal			
Awakening	12% DAVID (1955)	13%	27% KRISCHEK (1962)
Sleep	8% JANZ (1969)	18%	22% KRISCHEK (1962)
Diffuse	4% JANZ (1969)	6%	8% KRISCHEK (1962)
Psychomotor epilepsy	7% JANZ (1969)	18%	46% BAMBERGER and MATTHES (1959)
Cortical epilepsy	3% JANZ (1969)	5%	6% GIBBS and GIBBS (1952)

Table 22. Correlation between types of seizure in same individuals (males)

Type of seizure	Grand mal								Petit mal								Psycho-motor epilepsy		Cortical epilepsy		Number of diagnosis	
	A		S		D		O		West		Lennox		Absence		Myoclonic							
	n	exp	n	exp	n	exp	n	exp	n	exp	n	exp	n	exp	n	exp	n	exp	n	exp	to-tal	addi-tional
GM-A	84	-	3	11.4	3	10.8	0	-	1	0.2	3	1.1	22	7.5	13	3.7	8	14.0	2	6.3	139	55
-S		8.5	53	-	5	5.1	0	-	0	0.1	0	0.5	3	3.6	1	1.7	16	6.6	1	2.9	82	29
-D		9.6		6.1	50	-	0	-	0	0.1	0	0.6	4	4.0	2	1.9	17	7.4	2	3.3	83	33
-O		-		-		-	45	-	0	0.1	0	0.4	1	3.2	1	1.6	8	6.0	4	2.7	59	14
PM-West		0.4		0.3		C.3		0.2	2	-	1	0	0	0.2	0	0.1	0	0.3	0	0.2	4	2
-Lennox		0.9		0.5		C.5		0.5		0	2	-	0	0.4	0	0.2	0	0.7	0	0.3	7	5
-Absence		8.7		5.5		5.1		4.6		0.1		0.5	35	-	3	1.8	2	6.7	1	3.0	71	36
-Myoclonic		5.0		3.2		3.0		2.7		0.1		0.3		2.1	19	-	1	3.9	1	1.7	40	21
Psychomotor epilepsy		14.5		9.1		8.6		7.8		0.2		0.9		6.0		2.9	65	-	3	5.0	120	55
Cortical epilepsy		3.3		2.1		2.0		1.8		0		0.2		1.4		0.7		2.5	29	-	43	14

n: Observed number of patients with certain types of seizures.
exp: Expected number of patients.

Table 23. Correlation between types of seizure in same individuals (females)

Type of seizure	Grand mal A n	A exp	S n	S exp	D n	D exp	O n	O exp	Petit mal West n	West exp	Lennox n	Lennox exp	Absence n	Absence exp	Myoclonic n	Myoclonic exp	Psychomotor epilepsy n	exp	Cortical epilepsy n	exp	total	addi-tional
GM-A	63	–	2	9.6	3	8.5	0	–	0	0.5	0	0.5	23	9.3	11	4.3	10	14.4	1	2.9	113	50
-S		7.3	36	–	4	3.7	0	–	1	0.2	0	0.2	2	4.1	0	1.9	15	6.3	1	1.3	61	25
-D		7.2		4.1	32	–	0	–	0	0.2	0	0.2	5	4.0	0	1.8	12	6.2	1	1.3	57	25
-O		–		–		–	31	–	0	0.2	1	0.2	3	3.5	1	1.6	7	5.4	0	1.1	43	12
PM-West		0.2		0.1		0.1		0.1	1	–	0	0	0	0.1	0	0.1	0	0.2	0	0.1	2	0
-Lennox		0.7		0.4		0.3		0.3		0	3	–	0	0.4	1	0.2	0	0.6	1	0.1	6	4
-Absence		10.0		5.7		5.1		4.9		0.3		0.3	35	–	2	2.5	4	8.5	0	1.7	74	39
-Myoclonic		3.8		2.2		1.9		1.9		0.1		0.1		2.1	16	–	0	3.2	1	0.7	32	16
Psychomotor epilepsy		13.3		7.6		6.7		6.5		0.4		0.4		7.4		3.4	54	–	0	2.3	102	48
Cortical epilepsy		1.2		0.7		0.6		0.6		0		0		0.6		0.3		1.0	11	–	16	5

n: Observed number of patients with certain types of seizure.

exp: Expected number of patients.

Table 24. Correlation between main and additional types of seizure: relative coefficient of contingency

Type of seizure				
main	additional	Male	Female	Total
A-GM	S-GM	-.821	-.838	-.849
	D-GM	-.816	-.719	-.797
	Lennox syndrome	.333	-1.000	.072
	Absence PM	.498	.567	.543
	Myoclonic PM	.671	.589	.643
	Psychomotor epilepsy	-.634	-.359	-.555
	Cortical epilepsy	-.767	-.687	-.759
S-GM	D-GM	-.514	-.286	-.448
	Lennox syndrome	-1.000	-1.000	-1.000
	Absence PM	-.523	-.682	-.657
	Myoclonic PM	-.915	-1.000	-.830
	Psychomotor epilepsy	.114	.231	.162
	Cortical epilepsy	-.809	-.370	-.724
D-GM	Lennox syndrome	-1.000	-1.000	-1.000
	Absence PM	-.319	-.169	-.285
	Myoclonic PM	-.226	-1.000	-.636
	Psychomotor epilepsy	.179	.157	.168
	Cortical epilepsy	-.668	-.492	-.544
O-GM	Lennox syndrome	-1.000	.150	.000
	Absence PM	-.683	-.431	-.639
	Myoclonic PM	-.561	-.529	-.592
	Psychomotor epilepsy	.026	.023	.098
	Cortical epilepsy	-.174	-1.000	-.338
Lennox syndrome	Absence PM	-1.000	-1.000	-1.000
	Myoclonic PM	-1.000	.256	.001
	Psychomotor epilepsy	-1.000	-1.000	-1.000
	Cortical epilepsy	-1.000	.289	.000
Absence PM	Myoclonic PM	.029	-.184	.002
	Psychomotor epilepsy	-.748	-.592	-.693
	Cortical epilepsy	-.688	-1.000	-.820
Myoclonic PM	Psychomotor epilepsy	-.717	-1.000	-.876
	Cortical epilepsy	-.223	.000	-.143
Psychomotor epilepsy	Cortical epilepsy	-.532	-1.000	-.696

Table 25. Summary of characteristic findings in each type of seizure (%)

| | Grand mal | | | |
	A	S	D	O
Age (years)	15–24	45+	35+	5–24
%	40.8 ↑	23.6 ↑	37.8 ↑	46.1
Male %	57.1	59.6	61.0	59.2
Female %	42.9	40.4	39.0	40.8
Age at onset (years)	6–22	35+	0–4	5–14
%	77.6 ↑	22.5 ↑	18.3 ↑	36.8
EEG				
Paroxysmal	71.4 ↑	46.1 ↓	52.4 ↓	52.6
3/s sp–w–c	12.9 ↑	0 ↓	2.4	3.9
Atypical sp–w–c	20.4 ↑	1.1 ↓	4.9	10.5
2–2.5/s sp–w–c	4.8 ↑	0 ↓	2.4	1.3
3.5–5/s sp–w–c	9.5 ↑	1.1	1.2	5.3
Multiple sp–w–c	16.3 ↑	0 ↓	4.9	2.6
Temporal discharge	2.7	2.2	3.7	2.6
High voltage α-wave	14.3 ↑	– ↓ 6.4 –		7.9
β-EEG	20.4	10.1	12.2	15.8
Slow waves	35.4	39.3	35.4	38.2
Low voltage EEG	0.7	2.2	1.2	10.6
Hyperventilation change	42.2 ↑	11.2 ↓	24.4	28.9
Focal sign	6.8 ↓	16.9	19.5	14.5
Familial predisposition	10.9	6.7	˙7.3	7.9
Exogenous factors	7.5 ↓	6.7 ↓	15.9	18.4
Clinical association				
Positive	Abs			
	Myoc			
Negative	S–GM	A–GM	A–GM	
	D–GM	Lennox	Lennox	
		Abs	Myoc	
	Cort	Myoc	Cort	
		Cort		

↑ or ↓ = statistically significant increase or decrease. See text.

Abs = absence petit mal; Myoc = myclonic; Psm = psychomotor; Cort = cortical.

Petit mal				Psychomotor epilepsy	Cortical epilepsy	Total
Lennox	Absence	Myoclonic	Total			
5-24	5-24	10-39	5-29	50+	15-34	5-24
100.0	82.9 ↑	100.0 ↑	71.7 ↑	15.1	60.0	42.9
40.0	50.0	54.3	50.9	54.5	72.5	59.2
60.0	50.0	45.7	49.1	45.4	27.5	40.8
0-4	5-17	10-16	5-17	0-5,20-29	5-14	0-4,5-9
85.7	82.9 ↑	71.4 ↑	79,2 ↑	21.0↑,25.2↑	37.5	1o.7,17.2
100.0	72.9 ↑	82.9 ↑	77.4 ↑	66.4	60.0	59.2
0	18.6 ↑	17.1 ↑	16.0 ↑	1.7 ↓	2.5	5.1
60.0	18.6 ↑	31.4 ↑	27.4 ↑	5.9 ↓	5.0	11.2
20.0	5.7	5.7	6.6 ↑	0.8	2.5	2.1
20.0	11.4 ↑	11.4	12.3 ↑	0.8 ↓	2.5	5.4
20.0	18.6 ↑	17.1	19.8 ↑	1.7 ↓	2.5	7.1
0	4.3	0	3.8	9.2 ↑	5.0	3.6
0	12.8	14.3	13.3	10.9	0	10.1
0	21.4	40.0 ↑	26.4 ↑	18.5	25.0	17.4
80.0	38.6	22.9	37.7	37.8	27.5	36.3
0	0	0	0	2.5	7.5	3.0
40.0	51.4 ↑	60.0 ↑	51.9 ↑	20.2 ↓	30.0	30.5
40.0	5.7	5.7	7.5 ↓	30.3 ↑	32.5 ↑	15.5
20.0	21.4 ↑	11.4	17.9 ↑	6.7	10.0	9.9
0	2.9 ↓	11.4	6.6 ↓	9.2	32.5 ↑	12.9
	A-GM	A-GM				
S-GM	S-GM	S-GM		A-GM	A-GM	
D-GM	Psm	D-GM		Lennox	S-GM	
Abs	Cort	Psm		Abs	D-GM	
Psm				Myoc	Abs	
				Cort	Psm	

Table 26. Comparison among patients with pure awakening grand mal, absence petit mal, and myoclonic petit mal

Patient groups	Patients with pure awakening grand mal (N=53)		Patients with all Absence PM (N=70)		Patients with all myoclonic PM (N=35)	
	n	%	n	%	n	%
Male patients	33	62.3	35	50.0	19	54.3
Female patients	20	37.7	35	50.0	16	45.1
Age at onset (years)						
0- 9	5	9.4	< 42[a]	60.0	3	8.6
10-19	24	45.3	24	34.3	< 28	80.0
20-39	21	39.6	4	5.7	4	11.4
40+	3	5.7	> 0	–	> 0	–
EEG						
Paroxysmal	36	67.9	51	72.9	29	82.9
3/s sp-w-c	2	3.8	< 13	18.6	6	17.1
High voltage α-wave	8	15.1	9	12.9	5	14.3
β-EEG	9	17.0	15[b]	21.4	< 14	40.0
Slow waves	16	30.2	27	38.6	8	22.9
Low voltage EEG	0	–	0	–	0	–
Hyperventilation change	19	35.8	36	51.4	< 21	60.0
Focal sign	2	3.8	4	5.7	2	5.7
Familial predisposition	7	13.2	15	21.4	4	11.4
Exogenous factors	6	11.3	2	2.9	4	11.4

A statistically significant difference was noted when patients with absence PM and those with myoclonic PM was compared with patients with awakening grand mal.

[a]This was increased when compared with patients with myoclonic petit mal.
[b]This was decreased when compared with patients with myoclonic petit mal.

Table 27. Comparison among patients with grand mal of awakening, during sleep, diffuse, and occasional types

Types of seizure	Awakening (N=147)		Sleep (N=89)		Diffuse (N=82)		Occasional (N=76)	
	n	%	n	%	n	%	n	%
Male patients	84	57.1	53	59.6	50	61.0	45	59.2
Female patients	63	42.9	36	40.4	32	39.0	31	40.8
Age at onset (years)								
0– 9	43	29.3	> 18	20.2	> 27	32.9	> 17	22.4
10–19	70	47.6	32	36.0	22	26.8	22	28.9
20–39	29	19.7	< 25	28.1	< 28	34.1	< 32	42.1
40+	5	3.4	14	15.7	5[b]	6.1	5	6.6
EEG								
Paroxysmal	105	71.4	> 41	46.1	> 43	52.4	> 40	52.6
sp-w-c	48	32.7	> 1[a]	1.1	> 6	7.3	> 11	14.5
High voltage α-wave	21	14.3	> 4	4.5	7	8.5	6	7.9
β-EEG	30	20.4	> 9	10.1	10	12.2	12	15.8
Slow waves	52	35.4	35	39.3	29	35.4	29	38.2
Low voltage EEG	1	0.7	2	2.2	1	1.2	8	10.5
Hyperventilation change	62	42.2	> 10[a]	11.2	> 20[b]	24.4	22	28.9
Focal sign	10	6.8	< 15	16.9	< 16	19.5	11	14.5
Familial predisposition	16	10.9	6	6.7	6	7.3	6	7.9
Exogenous factors	11	7.5	6[a]	6.7	13	15.9	< 14	18.4

Only the statistically significant differences in three groups of patients with S-GM, D-GM, and O-GM, in comparison with awakening grand mal are noted by greater than or less than signs (> or <).

[a] Patients with S-GM revealed a decreased frequency when compared with those with occasional grand mal.

[b] Patients with D-GM showed a decreased or increased frequency when compared with those with grand mal during sleep.

Table 28. Comparison among patients with three types of seizure: pure grand mal, of awakening, during sleep and diffuse types

Pure type of seizure	Awakening (N=53)		Sleep (N=39)		Diffuse (N=31)		Total (N=123)	
	n	%	n	%	n	%	n	%
Male patients	33	62.3	27	69.2	21	67.7	81	65.9
Female patients	20	37.7	12	30.8	10	32.3	42	34.1
Age at onset (years)								
0- 9	5	9.4	7	17.9	5	16.1	17	13.8
10-19	24	45.3	16	41.0	10	32.3	50	40.7
20-39	21	39.6	10	25.6	12	38.7	43	34.9
40+	3	5.7	6	15.4	4	12.9	13	10.6
EEG								
Paroxysmal	36	67.9	> 14	35.9	> 13	41.9	63[b]	51.2
3/s sp-w-c	2	3.8	0	-	2	6.5	4	3.3
High voltage α-wave	8	15.1	1[a]	2.6	4	12.9	13	10.6
β-EEG	9	17.0	1[a]	2.6	5	16.1	15	12.2
Slow waves	16	30.2	16	41.0	10	32.3	42	34.1
Low voltage EEG	1	1.9	1	2.6	1	3.2	3	2.4
Hyperventilation change	19	35.8	> 5	12.8	10	32.3	34	27.6
Focal sign	2	3.8	3	7.7	5	16.1	10	8.1
Familial predisposition	7	13.2	4	10.3	1	3.2	12	9.8
Exogenous factors	6	11.3	4	10.3	5	16.1	15	12.2

A statistically significant difference was observed in patients with S-GM or D-GM compared with those with awakening grand mal as indicated by >.

[a]This was a statistically significantly decrease when compared with total patients with A-GM and D-GM.

[b]This was a statistically significantly decrease when compared with total patients without pure type of grand mal.

Table 29. Comparison between patients with combined petit mal and those with uncombined petit mal

Patient groups	Patients with uncombined PM (N=16)		Patients with combined PM (N=90)		Total patients with PM (N=106)	
	n	%	n	%	n	%
Male patients	8	50.0	46	41.1	54	50.9
Female patients	8	50.0	44	48.9	52	49.1
Age at onset (years)						
0- 4	4	25.0	11	12.2	15	14.2
5- 9	7	43.8	33	36.7	40⎫	37.7
10-14	2	12.5	27	30.0	29⎬↑	27.4
15-19	2	12.5	13	14.4	15⎭	14.2
20+	1	6.3	6	6.7	7	6.6
EEG						
Paroxysmal	11	68.8	71	78.9	82 ↑	77.4
3/s sp-w-c	0	-	< 17	18.9	17 ↑	16.0
Atypical sp-w-c	5	31.3	22	24.4	27 ↑	25.5
High voltage α-wave	2	12.5	12	13.3	14	13.2
β-EEG	7	43.8	21	23.3	28 ↑	26.4
Slow waves	7	43.8	33	36.7	40	37.7
Low voltage EEG	0	-	0	-	0	-
Hyperventilation change	9	56.3	46	51.1	55 ↑	51.9
Focal sign	1	6.3	7	7.8	8 ↓	7.5
Familial predisposition	3	18.8	16	17.8	19 ↑	17.9
Exogenous factors	2	12.5	5	5.6	7 ↓	6.6

The less-than sign (<) means the difference is statistically significant. Total petit mal patients showed the difference (↑ increase, ↓ decrease) compared with the rest of total patients.

Table 30. Comparison among patients with pure psychomotor and combined psychomotor epilepsy, pure grand mal during sleep, and diffuse grand mal

Patient groups	Patients with pure psychomotor epilepsy (N=24)		Patients with combined psychomotor epilepsy (N=95)		Patients with pure grand mal during sleep (N=39)		Patients with pure diffuse grand mal (N=31)	
	n	%	n	%	n	%	n	%
Male patients	15	62.5	50	52.5	27	69.2	21	67.7
Female patients	9	37.5	45	47.5	12	30.8	10	32.3
Age at onset (years)								
0- 9	8	33.3	28	29.5	7	17.9	5	16.1
10-19	5	20.8	25	26.3	16	41.0	10	32.3
20-39	8	33.3	33	34.7	10	25.6	12	38.7
40+	3	12.5	9	9.5	6	15.4	4	12.9
EEG								
Paroxysmal	17	70.8	62	65.3	> 14	35.9	> 13	41.9
sp-w-c	2	8.3	0	-	0	-	2	6.5
temporal discharge	3	12.5	8	8.4	0	-	1	3.2
β-EEG	9	37.5	> 13	13.7	> 1	2.6	5	16.1
Slow waves	9	37.5	36	37.9	16	41.0	10	32.3
Low voltage EEG	1	4.2	2	2.1	1	2.6	1	3.2
Hyperventilation change	6	25.0	18	18.9	5	12.8	10	32.5
Focal sign	6	25.0	30	31.6	3	7.7	5	16.1
Familial predisposition	2	8.3	6	6.3	4	10.3	1	3.2
Exogenous factors	2	8.3	9	9.5	4	10.3	5	16.1

A greater-than sign (>) indicates a statistically significant difference compared with patients with pure psychomotor epilepsy, three patient groups with combined psychomotor epilepsy, with pure grand mal during sleep and those with pure diffuse grand mal.

Table 31. Correlation between the age at onset of seizure and paroxysmal EEG

Age at onset (years)	Male							Female		
		3/s sp-w-c		Atypical sp-w-c		Paroxys-mal			3/s sp-w-c	
	N	n	%	n	%	n	%	N	n	%
0- 1	14	1	7.1	3	21.4	11	78.6	6	0	-
2- 4	15	2	13.1	1	6.7	10	66.7	15	2	13.3
5- 9	38	4	10.5	4	10.5	25	65.8	42	5	11.9
10-14	58	3	5.2	8	13.8	34	58.6	42	5	11.9
15-19	39	1	2.6	3	7.7	19	48.7	24	0	-
20-24	34	1	2.9	2	5.9	20	58.8	16	0	-
25-29	20	0	-	0	-	10	50.0	16	0	-
30-34	23	0	-	0	-	11	47.8	9	0	-
35-39	10	0	-	0	-	7	70.0	9	0	-
40-	25	0	-	1	4.0	10	40.0	11	0	-
Total	276	12	4.3	22	8.0	157	56.9	190	12	6.3

Table 32. Correlation between age at onset of seizure and α-EEG

Age at onset (years)	Male							Female		
		normal α		high-voltage α		no α			normal α	
	N	n	%	n	%	n	%	N	n	%
0- 1	14	11	78.6	1	7.1	2	14.3	6	2	33.3
2- 4	15	10	66.7	3	20.0	2	13.3	15	12	80.0
5- 9	38	32	84.2	3	7.9	3	7.9	42	30	71.4
10-14	58	44	75.9	5	8.6	9	15.5	42	30	71.4
15-19	39	36	92.3	1	2.6	2	5.3	24	18	75.0
20-24	34	31	91.2	1	2.9	2	5.9	16	9	56.2
25-29	20	19	95.0	0	-	1	5.0	16	11	68.8
30-34	23	16	69.6	3	13.0	4	17.4	9	8	88.9
35-39	10	10	100.0	0	-	0	-	9	6	66.7
40-	25	23	92.0	2	8.0	0	-	11	10	90.9
Total	276	232	84.1	19	6.9	25	9.0	190	136	71.6

patterns

Female				Total							
Atypical sp-w-c		Paroxys-mal			3/s sp-w-c		Atypical sp-w-c		Paroxys-mal	
n	%	n	%	N	n	%	n	%	n	%
3	50.0	5	83.3	20	1	5.0	6	30.0	16	80.0
4	26.7	12	80.0	30	4	13.3	5	16.7	22	73.3
7	16.7	29	69.0	80	9	11.3	11	13.8	54	67.5
6	14.3	29	69.0	100	8	8.0	14	14.0	63	63.0
6	25.0	14	58.3	63	1	1.6	9	14.3	33	52.4
2	12.5	11	68.8	50	1	2.0	4	8.0	31	62.0
1	6.3	5	31.3	36	0	-	1	2.8	15	41.7
0	-	4	44.4	32	0	-	0	-	15	46.9
0	-	6	66.7	19	0	-	0	-	13	68.4
1	9.1	4	36.4	36	0	-	2	5.6	14	38.9
30	15.8	119	62.6	466	24	5.2	52	11.2	276	59.2

Female				Total							
high-voltage α		no α			normal α		high-voltage α		no α	
n	%	n	%	N	n	%	n	%	n	%
2	33.3	2	33.3	20	13	65.0	3	15.0	4	20.0
1	6.7	2	13.3	30	22	73.4	4	13.3	4	13.3
5	11.9	7	16.7	80	62	77.5	8	10.0	10	12.5
7	16.7	5	11.9	100	74	74.0	12	12.0	14	14.0
3	12.5	3	12.5	63	54	85.7	4	6.3	5	8.0
5	31.3	2	12.5	50	40	80.0	6	12.0	4	8.0
4	25.0	1	6.2	36	30	83.3	4	11.1	2	5.6
0	-	1	11.1	32	24	75.0	3	9.4	5	15.6
0	-	3	33.3	19	16	84.2	0	-	3	15.8
1	9.1	0	-	36	33	90.9	3	9.1	0	-
28	14.7	26	13.7	466	368	79.0	47	10.1	51	10.9

Table 33. Correlation between age at onset of seizure and β-EEG

Age at onset (years)	Male			Female			Total		
	N	n	%	N	n	%	N	n	%
0- 1	14	1	7.1	6	0	-	20	1	5.0
2- 4	15	1	6.7	15	2	13.3	30	3	10.0
5- 9	38	9	23.7	42	12	28.6	80	21	26.3
10-14	58	8	13.8	42	11	26.2	100	19	19.0
15-19	39	5	12.8	24	8	33.3	63	13	20.6
20-24	34	4	11.8	16	4	25.0	50	8	16.0
25-29	20	2	10.0	16	4	25.0	36	6	16.7
30-34	23	3	13.0	9	0	-	32	3	9.4
35-39	10	2	20.0	9	1	11.1	19	3	15.8
40-	25	3	12.0	11	1	9.1	36	4	11.1
Total	276	38	13.8	190	43	22.6	466	81	17.4

Table 34. Correlation between age at onset of seizure and incidence of θ and θ-δ waves

Age at onset (years)	Male					Female					Total							
	N	θ-wave		θ-δ-wave		N	θ-wave		θ-δ-wave		N	θ-wave		θ-δ-wave		Total θ + δ waves	
		n	%	n	%		n	%	n	%		n	%	n	%	n	%
0- 1	14	2	14.3	4	28.6	6	2	33.3	3	50.0	20	4	20.0	7	35.0	11	55.0
2- 4	15	4	26.7	6	40.0	15	3	20.0	4	26.7	30	7	23.3	10	33.3	17	56.7
5- 9	38	12	31.6	8	21.1	42	11	26.2	8	19.0	80	23	28.8	16	20.0	39	48.8
10-14	58	13	22.4	13	22.4	42	7	16.7	5	11.9	100	20	20.0	18	18.0	38	38.0
15-19	39	4	10.3	5	12.8	24	6	25.0	4	16.7	63	10	15.8	9	14.3	19	30.2
20-24	34	5	14.7	5	14.7	16	3	18.8	2	12.5	50	8	16.0	7	14.0	15	30.0
25-29	20	5	25.0	4	20.0	16	4	25.0	0	-	36	9	25.0	4	11.1	13	36.1
30-34	23	4	17.4	0	-	9	2	22.2	2	22.2	32	6	18.8	2	6.3	8	25.0
35-39	10	1	10.0	1	10.0	9	2	22.2	0	-	19	3	15.8	1	5.3	4	21.1
40-	25	2	8.0	0	-	11	2	18.2	1	9.1	36	4	11.1	1	2.8	5	13.9
Total	276	52	18.8	46	16.7	190	42	22.1	29	15.3	466	94	20.2	75	16.1	169	36.3

Table 35. Correlation between the age at onset of seizure and familial predisposition

Age at onset (years)	Male			Female			Total		
	N	n	%	N	n	%	N	n	%
0- 1	14	3	21.4	6	1	16.7	20	4	20.0
2- 4	15	3	20.0	15	2	13.3	30	5	16.7
5- 9	38	3	7.9	42	7	16.7	80	10	12.5
10-14	58	11	19.0	42	3	7.1	100	14	14.0
15-19	39	6	15.4	24	1	4.2	63	7	11.1
20-24	34	O	-	16	1	6.3	50	1	2.0
25-29	20	2	10.0	16	1	6.3	36	3	8.3
30-34	23	O	-	9	O	-	32	O	-
35-39	10	1	10.0	9	O	-	19	1	5.3
40-	25	1	4.0	11	O	-	36	1	2.8
Total	276	30	10.9	190	16	8.4	466	46	9.9

Table 36. Correlation between the age at onset of seizure and exogenous
factors

Age at onset (years)	Male			Female			Total		
	N	n	%	N	n	%	N	n	%
0- 1	14	4	28.6	6	1	16.7	20	5	25.0
2- 4	15	2	13.3	15	1	6.7	30	3	10.0
5- 9	38	6	15.8	42	4	9.5	80	10	12.5
10-14	58	2	3.4	42	0	-	100	2	2.0
15-19	39	6	15.4	24	1	4.2	63	7	11.1
20-24	34	7	20.6	16	2	12.5	50	9	18.0
25-29	20	6	30.0	16	O	-	36	6	16.7
30-34	23	8	34.8	9	O	-	32	8	25.0
35-39	10	4	40.0	9	2	22.2	19	6	31.6
40-	25	3	12.0	11	1	9.1	36	4	11.1
Total	276	48	17.4	190	12	6.3	466	60	12.9

Table 37. Early, teen-age, middle-age, and late onset of epilepsy

Age at onset (years)	Early 0-9 (N=130)		Teen-age 10-19 (N=163)		Middle-age 20-39 (N=137)		Late 40+ (N=36)		Total (N=466)	
	n	%	n	%	n	%	n	%	n	%
Male patients	67	51.5	97	59.5	87	63.5	25	69.4	276	59.2
Female patients	63	48.5	66	40.5	50	36.5	11	30.6	190	40.8
Type of seizure										
Grand mal										
Awakening	43	33.1	70 ↑	42.9 >	29	21.2	5 ↓	13.9	147	31.5
Sleep	18	13.8	32	19.6	25	18.2 <	14 ↑	38.9	89	19.1
Diffuse	27	20.8	22	13.5	28	20.4	5	13.9	82	17.6
Occasional	17	13.1	22	13.5	32	23.4	5	13.9	76	16.3
Total	100	76.9	139	85.3	107	78.1	29	80.6	375	80.5
Petit mal										
West syndrome	3	2.3	0	-	0	-	0	-	3	0.6
Lennox syndrome	5	3.8	0	-	0	-	0	-	5	1.1
Absence	42 ↑	32.3 >	24	14.7 >	4 ↓	2.9	0 ↓	-	70	15.0
Myoclonic	9	6.9	23	14.1 >	3 ↓	2.2	0 ↓	-	35	7.5
Total	55 ↑	42.3 >	44	27.0 >	7 ↓	5.1	0 ↓	-	106	22.7
Psychomotor epilepsy	36	27.7	30 ↓	18.4 <	41	29.9	12	33.3	119	25.5
Cortical epilepsy	14	10.8	14	8.6	10	7.3	2	5.6	40	8.6
EEG										
Paroxysmal	92 ↑	70.8 >	96	58.9	74	54.0	14 ↓	38.9	276	59.2
Sp-w-c	36 ↑	27.7	32	19.6	6 ↓	4.4	2 ↓	5.6	76	16.3
Abnormal	73 ↑	56.2	74	45.4	52	38.0	9 ↓	25.0	208	44.6
High voltage α-wave	15	11.5	16	9.8	13	9.5	3	8.3	47	10.1
β-EEG	25	19.2	32	19.6	20	14.6	4	11.1	81	17.4
Slow waves	67 ↑	51.5 >	57	35.0	40	29.2 >	5 ↓	13.9	169	36.3
Low voltage EEG	1	0.8	2	1.2 <	10	7.3	0	-	13	2.8
Hyperventilation change	58 ↑	44.6 >	52	31.9 >	27	19.7	5 ↓	13.9	142	30.5
Focal sign	24	18.5	18	11.0	26	19.0	4	11.1	72	15.5
Familial predisposition	19 ↑	14.6	21 ↑	12.9 >	5	3.6	1	2.8	46	9.9
Exogenous factors	18	13.8	9	5.5 <	29	21.2	4	11.1	60	12.9

Patients with certain age onset (four groups of early, teen-age, middle-age, and late onset) are compared with three patient groups with other age onset of seizure. A statistically significant difference was indicated by an arrow (↑ increase or ↓ decrease). Two adjacent patient groups were also compared. The statistically significant difference was indicated by greater or less than signs (> or <).

Table 38. Characteristic correlation between various factors

Factors	Sex ratio	Age (years)	Age at onset (years)	EEG	Familial predis-position	Exogenous factors
<u>Sex</u>	(-)	Females were younger	Females were earlier starting	Females: → normal α, high voltage α, β-EEG, sp-w-c specific, 3.5-5/s sp-w-c, multiple sp-w-c	-	-
<u>EEG</u>						
Paroxysmal	♂ = ♀	Maximum at 5-14(19), thereafter decreased	Minimum at 0-14(19), thereafter decreased	→ Low voltage EEG	-	-
Typical sp-w-c	< ♀	with age	with age	Low voltage EEG, focal sign, hyperventilation change	-	-
Atypical sp-w-c	♂ < ♀			Focal sign, normal α, high voltage α, slow waves, hyperventilation change	↑	-
Normal α-wave	♂ > ♀	↗	↗	→ Sp-w-c	-	-
High voltage α-wave	♂ < ♀	↗	8-14 ↑	→ β, slow waves, sp-w-c	-	-
β-EEG	♂ < ♀	10-39 ↑	5-19 ↑	Normal α, high voltage α, High voltage s-w burst, Sharp wave	-	-

Slow waves	δ = ♀	⊟ →↑ ⤴ ⊟ − δ	θ →↑ ⤴ θ − δ	Low voltage EEG hyperventilation change focal sign paroxysmal	−	−
Low voltage EEG	δ = ♀	20-49 ↑ ↗	20-39 ↑	Paroxysmal ↓ slow waves ↑	−	−
Hyperventilation change	< ♀	↗	↗	Paroxysmal ↑ specific typical sp-w-c atypical sp-w-c slow waves	−	−
Focal sign	δ = ♀	See text	35-39 ↑	Paroxysmal ↑ slow waves	−	↑
<u>Familial predisposition</u>	δ = ♀	10-19 ↑	0-14 ↑ ⤴	Normal EEG ↓ specific ↑ atypical sp-w-c	(−)	↓
<u>Exogenous factors</u>	δ = ♀	50+ ↓ 30-49 ↑	20-39 ↑ 〰	Focal sign ↑	↓	(−)

Arrows indicate statistically increase ↑, or decrease ↓, and increase or decrease with increasing age or age at onset (⤴〰).

δ ≷ ♀ = significant difference.

< ♀ = higher frequency in female patients.

− = no sifnificant difference.

Table 39. Correlation between paroxysmal EEG patterns and age, basic EEG

| | Males sp-w-c | | | | | |
| | | typical | | atypical | | paroxysmal | |
	N	n	%	n	%	n	%
Age (years)							
5- 9	7	0	-	1	14.3	7	100.0
10-14	25	2	8.0	4	16.0	19	76.0
15-19	34	2	5.9	6	17.6	21	61.8
20-24	54	4	7.4	3	5.6	24	44.4
25-29	35	1	2.9	4	11.4	17	48.6
30-34	34	3	8.8	2	5.9	22	64.7
35-39	32	0	-	1	3.1	19	59.4
40-44	24	0	-	0	-	12	50.0
45-49	11	0	-	0	-	5	45.5
50-54	9	0	-	0	-	4	44.4
55-59	4	0	-	1	25.0	2	50.0
60-64	3	0	-	0	-	2	66.7
65-	4	0	-	0	-	3	75.0
Total	276	12	4.3	22	8.0	157	56.9
EEG							
Normal α	232	10	4.3	15	6.5	131	56.5
High voltage α	19	2	10.5	3	15.8	11	57.9
no α	25	0	-	4	16.0	15	60.0
β-EEG	38	0	-	6	15.8	24	63.2
θ-waves	52	2	2.6	8	15.4	47	90.4
θ-δ-waves	46	3	6.5	5	10.9	29	63.0
Low voltage EEG	9	0	-	0	-	2	22.2
Pathologic hyperventilation change	83	11	13.3	18	21.7	74	89.2
Focal sign	44	0	-	1	2.3	33	75.0
Familial predisposition	30	3	10.0	7	23.3	20	66.7
Exogenous factors	48	2	4.2	3	6.2	28	58.3

rhythms, familial predisposition and exogenous factors

| | Females sp-w-c | | | | | | | Total sp-w-c | | | | | |
| | typical | | atypical | | paroxysmal | | | typical | | atypical | | paroxysmal | |
N	n	%	n	%	n	%	N	n	%	n	%	n	%
7	1	14.3	1	14.3	5	71.4	14	1	7.1	2	14.3	12	85.7
17	4	23.5	4	23.5	17	100.0	42	6	14.3	8	19.0	36	85.7
31	1	3.2	7	22.6	20	64.5	65	3	4.6	13	20.0	41	63.1
25	2	8.0	1	4.0	17	68.0	79	6	7.6	4	5.1	41	51.9
28	1	3.6	4	14.3	14	50.0	63	2	3.2	8	12.7	31	49.2
24	0	-	7	29.2	13	54.2	58	3	5.2	9	15.5	35	60.3
17	2	11.8	1	5.9	8	47.1	49	2	4.1	2	4.1	27	55.1
10	0	-	1	10.0	6	60.0	34	0	-	1	2.9	18	52.9
10	1	10.0	2	20.0	7	70.0	21	1	4.8	2	9.5	12	57.1
9	0	-	2	22.2	6	66.7	18	0	-	2	11.1	10	55.6
5	0	-	0	-	3	60.0	9	0	-	1	11.1	5	55.6
4	0	-	0	-	2	50.0	7	0	-	0	-	4	57.1
3	0	-	0	-	1	33.3	7	0	-	0	-	4	57.1
190	12	6.3	30	15.8	119	62.6	466	24	5.2	52	11.2	276	59.2
136	8	5.9	16	11.8	80	58.8	368	18	4.9	31	8.4	211	57.3
28	3	10.7	7	25.0	21	75.0	47	5	10.6	10	21.3	32	68.1
26	1	3.8	7	26.9	18	69.2	51	1	2.0	11	21.6	33	64.7
43	2	4.7	7	16.3	26	60.5	81	2	2.5	13	16.0	50	61.7
42	1	1.6	10	15.9	36	85.7	94	3	2.1	15	16.0	83	88.3
29	6	20.7	7	24.1	26	89.7	75	9	12.0	12	16.0	55	73.3
4	0	-	0	-	2	50.0	13	0	-	0	-	4	30.8
59	10	8.3	28	23.1	54	91.5	142	21	14.8	43	30.3	128	90.1
28	0	-	2	7.1	23	82.1	72	0	-	3	4.2	56	77.8
16	1	6.3	5	31.3	12	75.0	46	4	8.7	12	26.1	32	69.6
12	0	-	2	16.7	7	58.3	60	2	3.3	5	8.3	35	58.3

Table 40. Paroxysmal EEG abnormalities and type of seizure

EEG	Author	Number of patients	Type of seizure		
			Petit mal	Grand mal	Others
3/sp-w-c	JASPER and KERSCHMAN (1941)	77	-/62.3	-/85.7	
	FINLEY and DYNES (1942)	19	-/73.7		
	GIBBS et al. (1943)	246	-/81.3		
	LENNOX and DAVIS (1950)	200	44.5/-		PM+GM/psychomotor 55.5%
	HESS and NEUHAUS (1952)	47	-/55.3		
	SILVERMAN (1954)	24	45.8/62.5	25.0/50.0	
	CLARK and KNOTT (1955)	94	23.4/69.1	21.3/67.0	
	HAUGSTED and HÖNKE (1956)	83	-/68.7		
	GOTO (1957)	61	63.9/82.0	3.3/26.2	
	KUIJER (1957)	78	-/98.7		
	LUNDERVOLD et al. (1959)	46	19.6/76.1	8.7/54.3	
	DALBY (1969)	342	47.1/-	15.8/-	
	TSUBOI and CHRISTIAN (this study 1976)	24	0/79.2	8.3/54.2	
Slow (2-2.5/s) sp-w-c	LENNOX and DAVIS (1950)	200	8.5/-	28.0/-	Massive myoclonic (18.5%) PM+GM and/or psychomotor (26.0%)
	SILVERMAN (1954)	11	9.1/36.4	54.5/81.8	
	CLARK and KNOTT (1955)	53	9.4/-	18.9/-	PM+GM 50.9%
	GOTO (1957)	21	4.8/4.8	23.8/38.1	Myoclonic 14.3%; akinetic 28.6%
	TSUBOI and CHRISTIAN (1976)	10	0/70.0	20.0/100.0	

	Author	N			Type of seizure
Multiple sp-w-c	SILVERMAN (1954)	26	3.8/7.7	80.0/84.6	
	GOTO (1957)	16	6.3/18.8	12.5/56.3	Akinetic 38,5; myoclonic 6.3
	HORI (1959)	55	-/9.1	-/65.5	Myoclonic (49.1); psychomotor (16); myoclonic 10.2
	NIEDERMEYER (1966)	215	18.6/38.1	30.7/56.7	
	TSUBOI and CHRISTIAN (1976)	33	12.1/63.6	24.2/90.9	
Irregular sp-w-c	SILVERMAN (1954)	11	9.1/45.4	45.4/81.8	
	GOTO (1957)	58	3.4/8.6	27.6/69.0	Psychomotor 29.3
	TSUBOI and CHRISTIAN (1976)	21	14.3/61.9	14.3/81.0	
Total sp-w-c	SILVERMAN (1954)	114	13.2/26.3	52.6/70.2	
	CLARK and KNOTT (1955)	178	15.7/69.1	22.5/73.6	
	GOTO (1957)	150	33.3/47.5	21.3/56.0	psychomotor (19), akinetic (17), myoclonic (11)
	LUNDERVOLD et al. (1959)	363	5.0/41.9	17.1/77.7	Focal (39), Lennox (20)
	TAKASE (1960)	100	33.0/60.0	32.0/61.0	psychomotor (6), akinetic (6), myoclonic (2)
	MORITA (1960)	105	8.5/-	51/-	psychomotor (30), myoclonic (4), akinetic (2)
	DALBY (1969)	437	36.8/-	12.4/-	Focal (13), myoclonic (9), psychomotor (3)
	TSUBOI and CHRISTIAN (1976)	76	7.9/63.2	18.5/86.8	

The first figure under type of seizure indicates the frequency (%) of paroxysmal EEG abnormality in patients with a pure type of seizure, and the second the type in patients with combined types of seizures.

Table 41. Patients with and without paroxysmal EEG abnormalities

Patient group	Patients with paroxysmal abnormality (N=276)			Patients with no paroxysmal abnormality (N=190)	
	n	%		n	%
Male patients	157	56.9		119	62.6
Female patients	119	43.1		71	37.4
Age at onset (years)					
0- 9	92	33.3	>	38	20.0
10-19	96	34.8		67	35.3
20-39	74	26.8		63	33.2
40+	14	5.1	<	22	11.6
Type of seizure					
Grand mal					
Awakening	105	38.0	>	42	22.1
Sleep	41	14.9	<	48	25.3
Diffuse	43	15.6		39	20.5
Occasional	40	14.5		36	18.9
Total	218	79.0		157	82.6
Petit mal					
West syndrome	2	0.7		1	0.5
Lennox syndrome	5	1.8		0	-
Absence	51	18.5	>	19	10.0
Myoclonic	29	10.5	>	6	3.2
Total	82	29.7	>	24	12.6
Psychomotor epilepsy	79	28.6		40	21.1
Cortical epilepsy	24	8.7		16	8.4
EEG					
Very slow waves (θ-δ)	55	19.9	>	20	10.5
Hyperventilation change	128	46.4	>	14	7.4
Focal sign	56	20.3	>	16	8.4
Familial predisposition	32	11.6		14	7.4
Exogenous factors	35	12.7		25	13.2

Table 42. Comparison between patients with typical, atypical and total sp-w-c, no sp-w-c, and with sp-w-c at age over 30 years

Patient group	Typical sp-w-c (N=24)		Atypical sp-w-c (N=52)		Total sp-w-c (N=76)		No sp-w-c (N=390)		Patients with sp-w-c at age over 30 years (N=23)	
	n	%	n	%	n	%	n	%	n	%
Male patients	12	50.0	22	42.3	34	44.7	242	62.1	7	30.4
Female patients	12	50.0	30	57.7	42	55.3	148	37.9	16↑	69.6
Age at onset (years)										
0- 4	5	20.8	11	21.2	16	21.1	34	8.7	2↑	8.7
5- 9	9	37.5	11	21.2	20	26.3	60	15.4	9↑	39.1
10-14	8	33.3	14	26.9	22	28.9	78	20.0	4	17.4
15-19	1	4.2	9	17.3	10	13.2	53	13.6	3	13.0
20+	1	4.2	7	13.5	8↓	10.5	165	42.3	5	21.7
Type of seizure										
Grand mal										
Awakening	18	75.0	30	57.7	48↑	63.2	99	25.4	16↑	69.6
Sleep	0	-	1	1.9	1↓	1.3	88	22.6	0↓	-
Diffuse	2	8.3	4	7.7	6↓	7.9	76	19.5	2	8.7
Occoasional	1	4.2	2	3.8	3	3.9	73	18.7	3	13.0
Total	23	95.8	43	82.7	66	86.8	309	79.2	18	78.3
Petit mal										
West syndrome	0	-	2	3.8	2	2.6	1	0.3	0	-
Lennox syndrome	0	-	3	5.8	3↑	3.9	2	0.5	0	-
Absence	13	54.2 >	13	25.0	26↑	34.2	44	11.3	8↑	34.8
Myoclonic	6	25.0	11	21.2	17↑	22.4	18	4.6	5↑	21.7
Total	19	79.2 >	29	55.8	48↑	63.2	58	14.9	13↑	56.5
Psychomotor epilepsy	2	8.3	7	13.5	9↓	11.8	110	28.2	2↓	8.7
Cortical epilepsy	1	4.2	2	3.8	3	3.9	37	9.5	2	8.7
EEG										
β-EEG	2	8.3	13	25.0	15	19.7	66	16.9	6	26.1
High voltage α-wave	5	20.8	10	19.2	15↑	19.7	32	8.2	4	17.4
Slow waves	12	50.0	27	51.9	39↑	51.3	130	33.3	10	43.4
Hyperventilation change	21	87.5	43	82.7	64↑	84.2	78	20.0	19↑	82.6
Focal sign	0	-	3	5.8	3↓	3.9	69	17.7	0↓	-
Familial predisposition	4	16.7	12	23.1	16↑	21.1	30	7.7	7↑	30.4
Exogenous factors	2	8.3	5	9.6	7	9.2	53	13.6	1	4.3

Statistically significant difference is indicated by arrows (↑ increased or ↓ decrease). Greater-than sign indicates significant difference between two groups of patients with typical and with atypical sp-w-c.

Table 43. Patients with various basic EEG rhythms

Patient group	High-voltage α (N=47)		β-EEG (N=81)		Slow wave EEG (N=215)		Low-voltage EEG (N=13)		Normal α EEG (N=368)	
	n	%	n	%	n	%	n	%	n	%
Male patients	19	40.4	38	46.9	144	58.0	9	69.2	232	63.0
Female patients	28↑	59.6	43	53.1	71	42.0	4	30.8	136↓	37.0
Age at onset (years)										
0- 9	15	31.9	25	30.9	67↑	39.6	1	7.7	97	26.4
10-19	16	34.0	32	39.5	57	33.7	2	15.4	128	34.8
20-39	13	27.7	20	24.7	40	23.7	10↑	76.9	110	29.9
40+	3	6.4	4	4.9	5↓	3.0	0	–	33	9.0
Type of seizure										
Grand mal										
Awakening	21↑	44.7	30	37.0	52	30.8	1↓	7.7	111	30.2
Sleep	4↓	8.5	9↓	11.1	35	20.7	2	15.4	74	20.1
Diffuse	7↓	14.9	10	12.3	29	17.2	1	7.7	68	18.5
Occasional	6	12.8	12	14.8	29	17.2	8↑	61.5	58	15.8
Total	37	78.7	57	70.4	138	81.7	12	92.3	297	80.7
Petit mal										
West syndrome	0	–	1	1.2	3	1.8	0	–	1	0.3
Lennox syndrome	0	–	0	–	4	2.4	0	–	3	0.8
Absence	9	19.1	15	18.5	27	16.0	0	–	54	14.7
Myoclonic	5	10.6	14↑	17.3	8	4.7	0	–	26	7.1
Total	14	29.8	28↑	34.6	40	23.7	0↓	–	78	21.2
Psychomotor epilepsy	13	27.7	22	27.2	45	26.6	3	23.1	89	24.2
Cortical epilepsy	0	–	10	12.3	11	6.5	3	23.1	36	9.8
EEG										
Paroxysmal	32	68.1	50	61.7	138↑	81.7	4↓	30.8	211	57.3
Sp-w-c	15↑	31.9	14	17.3	39↑	23.1	0	–	49	13.3
Slow waves	14	29.8	21↓	25.9	–	–	10↑	76.9	119↓	32.3
Focal sign	7	14.9	10	12.3	31	18.3	0	–	56	15.2
Hyperventilation change	18	38.3	27	33.3	63↑	37.3	2	15.4	109	29.6
Familial predisposition	8	17.0	12	14.8	15	8.9	1	7.7	30	8.2
Exogenous factors	5	10.6	9	11.1	24	14.2	4	30.8	47	12.8

Figures with arrows show statistically significant differences (↑ increase, ↓ decrease), when compared with the rest of the total patients.

Table 44. Patients with focal EEG abnormality: a) on the left or right side, b) temporal or extratemporal area

Patient group	Focal EEG (N=72)		Side				Area			
			Left (N=51)		Right (N=21)		Temporal (N=54)		Extratemporal (N=18)	
	n	%	n	%	n	%	n	%	n	%
Male patients	44	61.1	31	60.8	13	61.9	31	57.4	13	72.2
Female patients	28	38.9	20	39.2	8	38.1	23	42.6	5	27.8
Age at onset (years)										
0- 9	24	33.3	19	37.3	5	23.8	18	33.3	6	33.3
10-19	18	25.0	13	25.5	5	23.8	14	25.9	4	22.2
20-39	26	36.1	16	31.4	10	47.6	19	35.2	7	38.9
40+	4	5.6	3	5.9	1	4.8	3	5.6	1	5.6
Area										
Temporal	54	75.0	40	78.4	14	66.7	-	-	-	-
Extratemporal	18	25.0	11	21.6	7	33.3	-	-	-	-
Type of seizure										
Grand mal										
Awakening	10↓	13.9	8	15.7	2	9.5	6	11.1	4	22.2
Sleep	15	20.8	14	27.5 >	1	4.8	15	27.8 >	0	-
Diffuse	16	22.2	8	15.7 <	8	38.1	12	22.2	4	22.2
Occasional	11	15.3	4	7.8 <	7	33.3	7	13.0	4	22.2
Total	49	68.1	32	62.7	17	81.0	38	70.4	11	61.1
Petit mal										
West syndrome	0	-	0	-	0	-	0	-	0	-
Lennox syndrome	2	2.8	2	3.9	0	-	2	3.1	0	-
Absence	4	5.6	3	5.9	1	4.8	3	5.6	1	5.6
Myoclonic	2	2.8	2	3.9	0	-	0	-	2	11.1
Total	8↓	11.1	7	13.7	1	4.8	5	9.3	3	16.7
Psychomotor epilepsy	36↑	50.0	27	52.9	9	42.9	32	59.3 >	4	22.2
Cortical epilepsy	13↑	18.1	10	19.6	3	14.3	7	13.0	6	33.3
EEG										
Paroxysmal	56↑	77.8	37	72.5	19	90.5	43	79.6	13	72.2
Sp-w-c	3↓	4.2	3	5.9	0	-	2	3.7	1	5.6
Slow waves	31	43.1	24	47.1	7	33.3	25	46.3	6	33.3
Familial predisposition	6	8.3	5	9.8	1	4.8	6	11.1	0	-
Exogenous factors	19↑	26.4	11	21.6	8	38.1	9	16.7 <	10	55.6

Table 45. Patients with and without familial predisposition and patients with and without exogenous factors

Patient group	Familal predisposition with (N=46) n	%	without (N=420) n	%	Exogenous factors with (N=60) n	%	without (N=406) n	%
Male patients	30	65.2	246	58.6	48	80.0 >	228	56.2
Female patients	16	34.8	174	41.4	12	20.0	178	43.8
Age at onset (years)								
0- 9	19	41.3 >	111	26.4	18	30.0	112	27.6
10-19	21	45.7	142	33.8	9	15.0 <	154	37.9
20-39	5	10.9 <	132	31.4	29	48.3 >	108	26.6
40+	1	2.2	35	8.3	4	6.7	32	7.9
Type of seizure								
Grand mal								
Awakening	16	34.8	131	31.2	11	18.3 <	136	33.5
Sleep	6	13.0	83	19.8	6	10.0 <	83	20.4
Diffuse	6	13.0	76	18.1	13	21.7	69	17.0
Total	34	73.9	341	81.2	42	70.0	333	82.0
Petit mal								
Absence	15	32.6 >	55	13.1	2	3.3 <	68	16.7
Myoclonic	4	8.7	31	7.4	4	6.7	31	7.6
Total	19	41.3 >	87	20.7	7	11.7 <	99	24.4
Psychomotor epilepsy	8	17.4	111	26.4	11	18.3	108	26.6
Cortical epilepsy	4	8.7	36	8.6	13	21.7 >	27	6.7
EEG								
Paroxysmal	32	69.6	244	58.1	36	60.0	240	59.1
Sp-w-c	16	34.8 >	60	14.3	7	11.7	69	17.0
Abnormal	27	58.7 >	181	43.1	32	53.3	176	43.3
High voltage α-wave	8	17.4	39	9.3	5	8.3	42	10.3
β-EEG	12	26.1	69	16.4	9	15.0	72	17.7
Slow waves	15	32.6	154	36.7	24	40.0	145	35.7
Low voltage EEG	1	2.2	12	2.9	4	6.7	9	2.2
Hyperventilation change	19	41.3	123	29.3	25	41.7 >	117	28.8
Focal sign	6	13.0	66	15.7	19	31.7 >	53	13.1
Familial predisposition	-	-	-	-	1	1.7 <	45	11.1
Exogenous factors	1	2.2 <	59	14.0	-	-	-	-

> or < = statistically significant difference.

References

ADAMS, A.: Studies on the flat electroencephalogram in man. Electroenceph. clin. Neurophysiol. 11, 35-41 (1959).

AICARDI, J., CHEVRIE, J.J.: Convulsive status epilepticus in infants and children. A study of 239 cases. Epilepsia (Amst.) 11, 187-197 (1970).

AJMONE MARSAN, C., ZIVIN, L.S.: Factors related to the occurrence of typical paroxysmal abnormalities in the EEG of epileptic patients. Epilepsia (Amst.) 11, 361-382 (1970).

ARIMA, M.: Studies on spike in relation to age in children of epilepsy. Brain Nerve (Tokyo) 11, 579-584 (1959).

AUCKLAND, N.L., COX, M., CRICHTON, J.U., DUNN, H.G.: Prospective study of EEGs in children of low birth weight. EEG clin. Neurophysiol. 24, 692 (1969).

BAMBERGER, P., MATTHES, A.: Anfälle im Kindesalter. Basel: Karger 1959.

BANCAUD, J.: L'épilepsie après 60 ans. Expérience d'un service de neuro-chirurgie foncitonelle. Sem. Hôp. Paris 46, 3138-3140 (1970).

BEAUSSART, M., BEAUSSART-BOULENGE, L.: Epilepsie et hérédité. Etude à partir d'une population de 3500 épileptiques. Lille Med. 14, 19-27 (1969).

BECK, M.: Häufigkeit und klinische Bedeutung von Spikes and Waves im EEG jenseits des 30. Lebensjahres. Diss. Heidelberg 1971.

BEYER, L., JOVANOVIC, U.J.: Elektroenzephalographische und klinische Korrelate bei Aufwachepileptikern mit besonderer Berücksichtigung der therapeutischen Probleme. Nervenarzt 37, 333-336 (1966).

BOLDYREV, A.J.: The nature of the first seizure in epilepsy, in children and adults. Zh. Nevropat. Psikhiat. 70, 902-906 (1970).

BONDUELLE, M., SALLOU, C., GUILLARD, J.: Etude de 51 dossiers d'épilepsie ayant débuté après 60 ans. Sem. Hôp. Paris 46, 3141-3144 (1970).

BOWER, B.D., JEAVONS, P.M. (1959): Cited in JANZ (1969).

BRIDGE, E.M.: Epilepsy and Convulsive Disorders in Children. New York-Toronto-London: McGraw Hill 1949.

BUENO, M., MADOZ, P., MARTINEZ LAGE, J.M.: Encefalopatia epileptica infantil con punto onda difusa lenta (sindrome de Lennox). Rev. esp. Pediat. 26, 193-204 (1970).

CALDERON, A., PAAL, G.: Focal changes and EEG in petit mal epilepsy. Electroenceph. clin. Neurophysiol. 9, 350-351 (1957).

CARNEY, L.R., HUDGINS, R.L., ESPINOSA, R.E., KLASS, D.W.: Seizures beginning after the age of 60. Arch. intern. Med. 124, 707-709 (1969).

CASTELLS, C., MENDILAHARSU, C.: La epilepsia mióclonica bilateral y consciente. Acta neurol. lat.-amer. 4, 23-25 (1958).

160

CAVAZZUTTI, G.B., CAPELLA, L., GATTI, G.: Evoluzione dell EEG epilettico dalla prima infanzia alla adolescenza. Riv. Neurol. 39, 575-584 (1971).
CHARLTON, M.H., MELLINGER, J.F.: Infantile spasm and hypsarrhythmia. Electroenceph. clin. Neurophysiol. 29, 413 (1970).
CHRISTIAN, W.: Bioelektrische Charakteristik tagesperiodisch gebundener Verlaufsformen epileptischer Erkrankungen. Dtsch. Z. Nervenheilk. 181, 413-444 (1960).
CHRISTIAN, W.: Schlaf-Wach-Periodik bei Schlaf- und Aufwach-Epilepsien. Nervenarzt 32, 266-275 (1961).
CHRISTIAN, W.: Klinische Elektroenzephalographie. Stuttgart: Thieme 1968.
CHURCHILL, J.A.: The relationship of epilepsy to breech delivery. Electroenceph. clin. Neurophysiol. 11, 1-12 (1959).
CLARK, E.C., KNOTT, J.R.: Paroxysmal wave and spike activity and diagnostic sub-classification. Electroenceph. clin. Neurophysiol. 7, 161-164 (1955).
COURJON, J., ARTRU, F., ZESKOV, P.: A propos des crises d'epilepsie apparaissant après 60 ans observées en clientèle de neurologie dans un service de neuro-chirurgie. Sem.Hôp. Paris 46, 3129-3132 (1970).
CURRIER, R.D., KOOI, K.A., SAIDMAN, L.J.: Prognosis of "pure" petit mal. A follow-up study. Neurology (Minneap.) 13, 959-967 (1963).
DALBY, M.A.: Epilepsy and 3 per second spike and wave rhythms. Acta neurol. scand. 45, suppl. 40 (1969).
DAVID, J.: L'épilepsie du réveil (à propos de 100 observations). Thèse, Lyon 1955.
DIEKER, H.: Untersuchungen zur Genetik besonders regelmäßiger hoher Alpha-Wellen im EEG des Menschen. Hum. Gen. 4, 189-216 (1967).
DOOSE, H.: Die Altersgebundenheit pathologischer EEG-Potentiale am Beispiel des kindlichen Petit mal. Nervenarzt 35, 72-79 (1964a).
DOOSE, H.: Das akinetische Petit mal. II. Verlaufsformen und Beziehungen zu den Blitz- Nick- Salaamkrämpfen und den Absencen. Arch. Psychiat. Z. f.d. ges. Neurol. 205, 637-654 (1964b).
DOOSE, H.: Das akinetische Petit mal. I. Das klinische und elektroenzephalographische Bild der akinetischen Anfälle. Arch. Psychiat. Z. f.d. ges. Neurol. 205, 625-636 (1964c).
DOOSE, H., GERKEN, H., LEONHARDT, R., VÖLZKE, E., VÖLZ, C.: Centrencephalic myoclonic-astatic petit mal: clinical and genetic investigations. Neuropädiatrie 2, 59-78 (1970).
Editorial: Temporal lobe epilepsy. Brit. med. J. 3, 320-321 (1971).
EEG OLOFSSON, O.: The development of the electroencephalogram in normal children and adolscents from the age of 1 through 21 years. Acta paediat. scand. 59, 3-46 (1970).
EEG OLOFSSON, O.: The development of the electroencephalogram in normal adolscents from the age of 16 through 21 years. Neuropädiatrie 3, 11-45 (1971).
EEG OLOFSSON, O., PETERSEN, I., SELLDEN, U.: The development of the electroencephalogram in normal children from the age of 1 through 15 years. Paroxysmal activity. Neuropädiatrie 2, 375-404 (1971).

FALCONER, M.A.: Genetic and related aetiological factors in temporal lobe epilepsy. A review. Epilepsia (Amst.) 12, 13-31 (1971).

FERNANDEZ SALAS, A., CHINCHILLA COOPER, M., CIRANO, P.M.: Epilepsia de inicio tardio. Acta med. Costarric. 12, 113-120 (1969).

FEUERSTEIN, J., WEBER, M., KURTZ, D., ROHMER, F.: Etude statistiquie des crises épileptiques apparaissant après l'age des 60 ans. Sem. Hôp. Paris 46, 3125-3128 (1970).

FINLEY, K.H., DYNES, J.B.: Electroencephalographic studies in epilepsy. Brain 65, 256-265 (1942).

FISCHER, H.: Symptomatische Epilepsie bei cerebralen Gefäßprozessen. Arch. Psychiat. Z. f.d. ges. Neurol. 199, 296-310 (1959).

FUJIMORI, B., TOSHIKATSU, Y., ISHIBASHI, Y., TAKEI, T.: Analysis of the elctroencephalogram of children by histogram method. Electroenceph. clin. Neurophysiol. 10, 241-252 (1958).

FURUICHI, Y.: Clinical and electroencephalographical study of nocturnal epilepsy. Psychiat. Neurol. jap. 71, 101-113 (1969).

FUSTER, B., CASTELLS, C., RODRIGUEZ, B.: Psychomotor attacks of subcortical origin. Arch. Neurol. Psychiat. (Chicago) 71, 466-472 (1954).

GABOR, A.J., AJMONE MARSAN, C.: Co-existence of focal and bilateral diffuse paroxysmal discharges in epileptics. Clinical-electrographic study. Epilepsia (Amst.) 10, 453-472 (1969).

GÄNSHIRT, H.: Schlaf-, Aufwach- und diffuse Epilepsien im Schlaf- und Wach-Elektroenzephalogramm. Nervenarzt 32, 130 (1961).

GÄNSHIRT, H.: Anfälle beim alten Menschen. Ärztl. Prax. 22, 4825-4827 (1970).

GÄNSHIRT, H., VETTER, K.: Schlafelektroenzephalogramm und Schlaf-Wachperiodik bei Epilepsien. Nervenarzt 32, 275-279 (1961).

GARCEZ DE SENA, P.: Epilepsia, conceito, incidencia e fatores patogenicos. Neurobiologia 32, 42-49 (1969).

GARSCHE, R.: Das Elektroenzephalogramm bei den psychomotorischen Anfällen im Kindesalter. Arch. Kinderheilk. 153, 27-54 (1956).

GARSCHE, R.: Die cerebralen "kleinen" Anfälle des Kindes. Anfallsmorphe, EEG und Differentialdiagnostik. Ergebn. inn. Med. Kinderheilk. 9, 228-281 (1958).

GASTAUT, H.: The Epilepsies. Electro-Clinical Correlations. Springfield, Ill.: Charles C. Thomas 1954.

GASTAUT, H.: Clinical and electro-encephalographic classification of epileptic seizures. Epilepsia (Amst.) 11, 102-113 (1970).

GASTAUT, H., ROGER, J., SOULAYROL, R., PINSARD, N.: L'encéphalopathie myoclonique infantile avec hypsarrhythmia (syndrome de West). Paris: Masson 1964.

GENTILE, G., MOMBELLI, A.M., BERGAMINI, L., RICCIO, A.: Studio longitudinale (5-17 anni) eletto clinico dell' encefalopatia epilettica dell'infanzia a punte onda lente diffuse (sindrome di Lennox). Riv. Pat. nerv. ment. 90, 173-177 (1969).

GIBBERD, F.B.: The prognosis of petit mal. Brain 89, 531-538 (1966).

GIBBERD, F.B.: Epilepsy. Brit. med. J. 4, 281-284 (1969).

GIBBS, E.L., FLEMING, M.M., GIBBS, F.A.: Diagnosis and prognosis of hypsarrhythmia and infantile spasm. Pediatrics 13, 66-73 (1954).

GIBBS, F.A., GIBBS, E.L.: Atlas of Electroencephalography. Cambridge, Mass.: Addison-Wesley Press 1952.

GIBBS, F.A., GIBBS, E.L., LENNOX, W.G.: EEG-classification of
   epileptic patients and control subjects. Arch. Neurol.
   Psychiat. 50, 111-128 (1943).
GLASER, G.H., DIXON, M.S.: Psychomotor seizures in childhood.
   A clinical study. Neurology (Minneap.) 6, 646-656 (1956).
GLASER, G.H., GOLUB, L.M.: The EEG of psychomotor seizures in
   childhood. Electroenceph. clin. Neurophysiol. 7, 329-340
   (1955).
GÖTZE, W., VOGEL, F., WOLSTER, M.: Findet man im Hirnstrombild
   von Zwillingen besonders häufig pathologische Veränderungen?
   Dtsch. Z. Nervenheilk. 177, 374-377 (1958).
GOMES LINS, S., FARIAS DA SILVA, W.: Estudo electro-clinico e
   terapeutico de 400 epilepticos com crises niniciadas entre
   10 e 15 anos. Neurobiologia 32, 119-132 (1969).
GOTO, Y.: The study on the correlation between spike and wave
   complex and clinical seizure pattern. Psychiat. Neurol. jap.
   59, 1071-1087 (1957).
GOWERS, W.: Epilepsy and Other Chronic Convulsive Diseases,
   Their Causes, Symptoms and Treatment. London: J.A. Churchill
   1901.
GREGORIADES, A.D.: A medical and social survey of 231 children
   with seizures. Epilepsia (Amst.) 13, 13-20 (1972).
HANSOTIA, P.: Petit mal: a critical review. Neurology (Bombay)
   17, 197-202 (1969).
HANSOTIA, P., WAIDIA, N.H.: Temporal lobe epilepsy with "ab-
   sences". Dis. nerv. Syst. 32, 316-319 (1971).
HARVALD, B.: Heredity in epilepsy. An EEG study of relatives of
   epileptics. Op. Ex. Dom. Biol. Hered. Hum. Univ. Hafn. 35,
   9-122 (1954).
HAUGSTED, H., HÖNKE, P.: Petit mal seizures and wave- and spike
   rhythms in epileptic children and adults. Acta psychiat. scand.
   Suppl. 108, 169-175 (1956).
HERTOFT, P.: The clinical, electroencephalographic and social
   prognosis in petit mal epilepsy. Epilepsia (Amst.) 4, 298-
   314 (1963).
HESS, R.: Verlaufsuntersuchungen über Anfälle und EEG bei klinischen Epilepsien. Arch. Psychiat. Z. f.d. ges. Neurol. 197,
   568-593 (1958).
HESS, R., BAUER, G., KETZ, E.: Centrencephale Epilepsie, tempo-
   rale Epilepsie: Entitäten oder Abstraktionen? Nervenarzt 41,
   525-529 (1970).
Hess, R., NEUHAUS, T.: Das Elektroenzephalogramm bei Blitz-,
   Nick- und Salaamkrämpfen und bei anderen Anfallsformen des
   Kindesalters. Arch. Psychiat. Z. f.d. ges. Neurol. 189, 37-
   58 (1952).
HILL, D.: EEG in episodic psychotic and psychopathic behavior;
   a classification of data. Electroenceph. clin. Neurophysiol.
   4, 419-442 (1952).
HOCKADAY, H.J.M., WHITTY, C.W.M.: Factors determining the electroencephalogram in migraine: A study of 560 patients according
   to clinical type of migraine. Brain 92, 769-788 (1969).
HOLOWACH, J., THURSTON, D.L., O'LEARY, J.L.: Petit mal epilepsy.
   Pediatrics 30, 893-901 (1962).
HOPKINS, H.: The time of appearance of epileptic seizures in
   relation to age, duration and type of the syndrome. J. nerv.
   ment. Dis. 77, 153-162 (1933).

HORI, H.: Correlation between clinical and electroencephalo-
   graphic findings regarding multiple spikes and multiple spikes-
   and-wave complex. Psychiat. Neurol. jap. 61, 1474-1485 (1959).
HUGHES, J.R.: EEG epileptiform abnormalities at different ages.
   Epilepsia (Amst.) 8, 93-104 (1967).
HYLLESTED, K., PAKKENBERG, H.: Prognosis in epilepsy of late
   onset. Neurology (Minneap.) 13, 641-644 (1963).
ISHIKURO, R.: Spikes and wave complex in the EEG and clinical
   pictures. Folia psychiat. neurol. jap. 11, 58-69 (1957).
JANZ, D.: "Diffuse" Epilepsien, als Ausdruck einer Verlaufsform
   vorwiegend symptomatischer Epilepsien im Vergleich zu "Nacht"-
   und "Aufwachepilepsien". Dtsch. Z. Nervenheilk. 170, 486-513
   (1953).
JANZ, D.: Anfallsbild und Verlaufsform epileptischer Erkrankungen.
   Nervenarzt 26, 20-28 (1955).
JANZ, D.: Die Epilepsien. Spezielle Pathologie und Therapie.
   Stuttgart: Thieme 1969.
JANZ, D., AKOS, R.: Über die Rolle pränataler Faktoren bei der
   Propulsiv-Petit-mal-Epilepsie (West-Syndrom). J. neurol. Sci.
   4, 401-406 (1967).
JANZ, D., CHRISTIAN, W.: Impulsiv-Petit mal. Dtsch. Z. Nerven-
   heilk. 176, 346-386 (1957).
JANZ, D., MATTHES, A.: Die Propulsiv-Petit mal-Epilepsie. Klinik
   und Verlauf der sog. Blitz-, Nick- und Salaamkrämpfe. Basel:
   Karger 1955.
JASPER, H., KERSCHMANN, J.: Electroencephalographic classification
   of the epilepsies. Arch. Neurol. Psychiat. (Chicago) 45, 903-
   943 (1941).
JASPER, H., PERTUISSET, B., FLANIGIN, H.: EEG and cortical elec-
   trograms in patients with temporal lobe seizures. Arch. Neurol.
   Psychiat. (Chicago) 65, 272-290 (1951).
JEAVONS, P.M., BOWER, B.D.: Infantile spasms. A review of the
   literature and a study of 122 cases. Clin. develop. Med. No.
   15, London 1964.
JELLIFFE, E.S., NETKIN, J.: The pyknolepsies. Amer. J. Psychiat.
   91, 679-692 (1934).
JERAS, J.: Temporallappenepilepsie bei Kindern. Zbl. ges. Neurol.
   Psychiat. 155, 238 (1960).
JERAS, J.: Psychomotor paroxysma in childhood. Zdrav. Vestn. 39,
   75-80 (1970).
JOVANOVIC, U.J.: Das Schlafverhalten der Epileptiker. 1. Schlaf-
   dauer, Schlaftiefe und Besonderheiten der Schlafperiodik.
   Dtsch. Z. Nervenheilk. 190, 159-198 (1967).
JUHASZ, P., HALSZ, P.: The relation of petit mal to partial and
   generalized epileptic mechanisms. Excerpta med. (Amst.) ICS
   193, 235 (1969).
JUNG, R.: Zur Klinik und Elektrophysiologie des "petit mal". 4.
   Congr. intern. d'EEG et Neurophysiol. clinique. Acta med.
   belg. Bruxelles 296 (1957).
JUNG, R.: Cited in JANZ (1969).
KARBOWSKI, K., VASELLA, F., SCHNEIDER, H.: Electroencephalographic
   aspects of Lennox syndrome. Europ. Neurol. 4, 301-311 (1970).
KELLAWAY, P.: Myoclonic phenomena in infants. Electroenceph.
   clin. Neurophysiol. 4, 243-244 (1952).
KRISCHEK, J.: Pneumoencephalographische Studien bei Epileptikern.
   Psychiat. et Neurol. (Basel) 138, 345-355 (1959).

KRISCHEK, J.: Die Schlaf-Wach-Periodik der Grand-mal-Epilepsie
und die sich daraus ergebenden therapeutischen Konsequenzen.
Dtsch. med. Wschr. 87, 2528-2533 (1962).

KRUSE, R.: Schlafepilepsie im Kindesalter. Grand mal und fokale
Anfälle. Klinik und EEG. Nervenarzt 35, 200-207 (1964).

KRUSE, R.: Das myoklonisch-astatische Petit mal. Berlin-Heidelberg-
New York: Springer-Verlag 1968.

KUHLO, W., SCHWARZ, J.: Katamnestische Untersuchungen bei soge-
nannter Spätepilepsie. Arch. Psychiat. Nervenkr. 215, 8-21
(1971).

KUIJER, A.S.: Clinical type of seizures associated with rhythmic
bilateral wave- and spikes. Observation in 78 cases. Electroenceph. clin. Neurophysiol. 9, 557 (1957).

LANCE, J.W.: Classification and treatment of myoclonus. Proc.
Austr. Ass. Neurol. 7, 61-64 (1969).

LANGDON-DOWN, M., BRAIN, W.R.: Time of day in relation to convulsions in epilepsy. Lancet (1929) I, 1029-1032.

LECASBLE, R.: Les myoclonies épileptiques. In: Bases physiolo-
giques et aspects cliniques de l'epilepsie. ALAUOUANINE, T.
(ed.). Paris: Masson 1958.

LEDER,A.: Aufwachepilepsie. Eine testpsychologische Untersuchung.
Bern: Huber 1969.

LENNOX, W.G., DAVIS, J.P.: Clinical correlates of the fast and
slow spike-wave EEG. Pediatrics 5, 626-644 (1950).

LENNOX, W.G., LENNOX, M.A.: Epilepsy and Related Disorders.
Boston: Little, Brown 1960.

LENNOX-BUCHTHAL, M.: Febrile and nocturnal convulsions in mono-
zygotic twins. Epilepsia (Amst.) 12, 147-156 (1971).

LESNY, I.: Evolution of the EEG changes in infantile spasms.
Electroenceph. clin. Neurophysiol. 30, 275 (1971).

LIVINGSTON, S.: The Diagnosis and Treatment of Convulsive Disorders in Children. Springfield, Ill.: Charles C Thomas 1954.

LIVINGSTON, S., TORRES, I., Pauli, L.L., RIDER, R.V.: Petit mal
epilepsy. Results of a prolonged follow-up study of 117 patients. J. Amer. med. Ass. 194, 227-232 (1965).

LOISEAU, P., BEAUSSART, M.: Hereditary factors in partial epilepsy. Epilepsia (Amst.) 10, 23-31 (1969).

LOISEAU, P., COHADON, S., FAURE, J.: Remarques sur un cas d'
épilepsie partielle continue. Rev. neurol. 108, 107-111 (1963).

LUNDERVOLD, A., HENRIKSEN, G.F., FEGERSTEN, L.: The spike and
wave complex; a clinical correlation. Electroenceph. clin.
Neurophysiol. 11, 13-22 (1959).

LUPU, I., MACOVEI-LUPU, M., COCINSCHI, R., FRATILA, A.: Febrile
infantile convulsions. Electro-clinical contributions. Electroenceph. clin. Neurophysiol. 30, 360-361 (1971).

MAGNUS, O., PENFIELD, W., JASPER, H.: Mastication and consciousness
in epileptic seizures. Acta psychiat. scand. 27, 91-99 (1952).

MATTHES, A.: Die psychomotorische Epilepsie im Kindesalter. Z.
Kinderheilk. 85, 455-471 (I), 472-492 (II), 668-685 (III)
(1961).

MATTHES, A.: Epilepsie im Kindesalter. Z. allg. Med. Landarzt
46, 451-456 (1970).

MATTHES, A., MALLMANN-MÜHLBERGER, E.: Die Propulsive-Petit-Mal-
Epilepsie und ihre Behandlung mit Hormonen. Dtsch. med. Wschr.
88, 426-434 (1963).

MATTHES, A., WEBER, H.-P.: Klinische und elektroenzephalographische Familienuntersuchungen bei Pyknolepsien. Dtsch. med.
Wschr. 93, 429-435 (1968).

MAYER, K., TRÜBESTEIN, G.: Über Ursachen und Verlaufsformen der sogenannten Spätepilepsie. Med. Welt 19, 1951-1956 (1968).

Medical World News: New research highlights in the possibility and clinical necessity of more specific treatment in epilepsy. Medical World News 11, 28-36 (1970).

MEYER-MICKELEIT, R.W.: Die Dämmerattacken als charakteristischer Anfallstyp der temporalen Epilepsie. Nervenarzt 24, 331-346 (1953).

MORITA, S.: Clinical evaluation of spike and wave-complex. Brain Nerve (Tokyo) 12, 117-125 (1960).

MUNDY-CASTLE, A.C.: Theta and beta rhythm in the EEG of normal adults. Electroenceph. clin. Neurophysiol. 3, 477-486 (1951).

NIEDERMEYER, E.: Psychomotor seizure with generalized synchronous spike and wave discharge. Electroenceph. clin. Neurophysiol. 6, 495-496 (1954).

NIEDERMEYER, E.: Concerning the problem of psychomotor epilepsy in childhood. Electroenceph. clin. Neurophysiol. 9, 350 (1957).

NIEDERMEYER, E.: Über Epilepsie im höheren Lebensalter. Arch. Psychiat. Z. f.d. ges. Neurol. 197, 248-262 (1958).

NIEDERMEYER, E.: The generalized multiple spike discharge. An electro-clinical study. Electroenceph. clin. Neurophysiol. 20, 133-138 (1966).

NIEDERMEYER, E.: The Lennox-Gastaut syndrome: a severe type of childhood epilepsy. Dtsch. Z. Nervenheilk. 195, 263-282 (1969).

NIEDERMEYER, E., WALTER, A.E., BURTON, C.: The slow spike-wave complex as a correlate of frontal and fronto-temporal post-traumatic epilepsy. Europ. Neurol. 3, 330-346 (1970).

NISHIURA, N.: A clinico-genetic and electroencephalographic study of epilepsy. Bull. Osaka med. Sch. 12, 59-82 (1966).

O'BRIEN, J.L., GOLDENSOHN, E.S., HOEFER, P.F.A.: Electroencephalographic abnormalities in addition to bilaterally synchronous 3 per second spike and wave activity in petit mal. Electroenceph. clin. Neurophysiol. 11, 747-761 (1959).

OHTAHARA, S., OKA, E., BAN, T.: The Lennox syndrome. Electroencephalographic study. Clin. Neurol. (Tokyo) 10, 617-625 (1970).

OTOMO, E., TSUBAKI, T.: Electroencephalography in subjects sixty years and over. Electroenceph. clin. Neurophysiol. 20, 77-82 (1966).

OUNSTED, C.: The factor of inheritance in convulsive disorders in childhood. Proc. roy. Soc. Med. 45, 865-868 (1952).

PAAL, G.: Follow-up and EEG studies in pyknolepsy. Electroenceph. clin. Neurophysiol. 9, 350 (1957).

PAAL, G.: Katamnestische Untersuchungen und EEG bei Pyknolepsie. Arch. Psychiat. Z. f.d. ges. Neurol. 196, 48-62 (1957).

PACHE, H.D.: Die Stellung der Pyknolepsie im cerebralen Anfallsgeschehen des Kindes. München: Habil. 1952.

PARTY, F.L.: The relation of time of day, sleep and other factors to the incidence of epileptic seizures. Amer. J. Psychiat. 10, 789 (1931).

PATRICK, H.T., LEVY, D.M.: Early convulsions in epileptics and others. J. Amer. med. Ass. 82, 375-384 (1924).

PAZZAGLIA, P., FRANK, L., ORIOLDI, G., LUGARESI, E.: L'evoluzione elettro clinica del piccolo male tipico. Riv. Neurol. 39, 557-566 (1969).

PAZZAGLIA, P., FRANK, L., ROGER, J., TASSEINARI, C.A., LUGARESI, E.: Prognosi e nosologia del piccolo male: Obervazioni su 175 casi. Riv. Neurol. 41, 265-273 (1971).

PEDERSEN, H.E., KROGH, E.: The prognostic consequences of familial predisposition and sex in epilepsy. Acta neurol. scand. 47, 106-116 (1971).

PENFIELD, W., JASPER, H.: Epilepsy and the Functional Anatomy of the Human Brain. Boston: Little, Brown 1954.

PETERSEN, I., EEG OLOFSSON, O.: The development of the electroencephalogram in normal children form the age of 1 through 15 years. Neuropädiatrie 2, 247-304 (1971).

PINE and PINE (1953): Cited in Götze et al. (1958).

POCH, G.F., DELAMONICA, E.A.: Encefalopatia mioclonica infantil hipsarritmica y esclerosis tuberosa. Pren. méd. argent. 56, 1271-1272 (1969).

POHLISCH, K.: Differential-Diagnose der genuinen und sogenannten traumatischen Epilepsie. Arch. Psychiat. Z. Neurol. 185, 466-473 (1950).

RAYNOR, R.B., PAINE, R.S., CARMICHAEL, F.R.: Epilepsy of late onset. Neurology (Minneap.) 9, 111-117 (1959).

RICCI, C.B., SCARINCI, A.: Clinical correlations and evolutions in epileptic EEG foci in children. Electroenceph. clin. Neurophysiol. 15, 919-920 (1963).

RICHTER, K.: EEG Untersuchungen von Angehörigen genuiner Epileptiker. Arch. Psychiat. Neurol. 194, 443-455 (1956).

ROBERT, F., KARBOWSKI, K.: Elektroenzephalographische Befunde bei Schulkindern. Helv. paediat. Acta 26, 286-299 (1971).

ROBIN, A.: Le démembrement des pycnolepsies de l'enfance et de l'adolescence. Acta neurol. belg. 9, 881-893 (1960).

ROBINSON, L., OSTERHELD, R.G.: The electro- encephalogram in epileptic patients aged five to 80 years. J. nerv. ment. Dis. 106, 464-470 (1947).

RODRIGO LONDONO, L.: Epidemiologia de la epilepsia. Neurocirugía 27, 21-33 (1969).

ROSENTHAL, C.: Der pyknoleptische Anfallstyp. Arch. Psychiat. Nervenheilk. 84, 511-513 (1928).

SACHS, B., HAUSMANN, L.: Nervous and Mental Disorders from Birth through Adolescence. New York: Paul B. Hoeber 1926.

SCHERMAN, R.G., ABRAHAM, K.: "Centrencephalic" electroencephalographic patterns in precocious puberty. Electroenceph. clin. Neurophysiol. 15, 559-567 (1963).

SCHNEIDER, H., VASSELLA, F., KARBOWSKI, K.: The Lennox syndrome. A clinical study of 40 children. Europ. Neurol. 4, 289-300 (1970).

SILVERMAN, A.J., BUSSE, E.W., BARNES, R.H.: Studies in the process of aging: Electroencephalographic findings in 400 elderly subjects. Electroenceph. clin. Neurophysiol. 7, 67-74 (1955).

SILVERMAN, D.: Clinical correlates of the spike-wave complex. Electroenceph. clin. Neurophysiol. 6, 663-669 (1954).

SIMONSON, H.: One-sided cerebral ventricular dilatation in cryptogenic epilepsy. Acta psychiat. scand. Suppl. 74 (1950).

SINDRUP, E.: Elektroenzephalographische Befunde bei Patienten psychomotorischer Epilepsie und Psychose. EEG EMG (Stuttgart) 1, 206 (1970).

SMITH, B., ROBINSON, G.C., LENNOX, W.G.: Acquired epilepsy (A study of 535 cases). Neurology (Minneap.) 4, 19-28 (1954).

SOMASUNDARAM, C.P., MATHAI, K.V., CHANDY, J.: A psychometric
study of patients with convulsive disorders. Neurology
(Bombay) 16, 155-158 (1969).
STÖGMANN, W.: Zur Epilepsie im Kindesalter. Wien. med. Wschr.
119, 845-849 (1969).
STÖGMANN, W., LORENZONI, E.: Nosologische Untersuchungen bei
Blitz-Nick-Salaam-Krämpfen. Wien. Z. Nervenheilk. 28, 1-11
(1970).
STRACKEE-KUIJER, A.: Clinical type of seizures associated with
rhythmic bilateral wave-and-spikes. Observation in 78 cases.
Electroenceph. clin. Neurophysiol. 9, 557 (1957).
SVATY, J., DIENSTBIEROVA, A.: The course (progress) of epilepsy
in 245 children in the time up to maturation, and the social
activities of young epileptics. (In Czech). Cse. Pediat. 24,
1086-1091 (1969).
TAEN, S., SUZUKI, M., GOTO, Y., MORI, O.: Clinico-statistical
observations on epilepsy. Brain Nerve (Tokyo) 8, 509-514
(1956).
TAKAHASHI, T., NIEDERMEYER, E., KNOTT, J.R.: The EEG in older
and younger adult groups with convulsive disorder. Epilepsia
(Amst.) 6, 24-32 (1965).
TAKASE, K.: Clinical studies of the spike and wave complex.
Brain Nerve (Tokyo) 12, 305-321 (1960).
TAYLOR, D.C.: Differential rates of cerebral maturation between
sexes and between hemispheres. Evidence from epilepsy. Lancet
(1969) II, 140-142.
THIERFELDER, F.: Die klinischen Erscheinungsformen hereditärer
Epilepsien. Diss. Heidelberg 1953.
TOURNIER, G., LELORD, G., RÉMOND, A.: A study of electro-clinical
correlations in the epileptic sequels of the infectious
meningoencephalitides. Electroenceph. clin. Neurophysiol. 7,
450 (1955).
TÜKEL, K., JASPER, H.: The EEG in parasagittal lesions. Electroenceph. clin. Neurophysiol. 4, 481-494 (1952).
VERCELETTO, P., DELOBEL, R.: Etude des facteurs étiologiques
et prognostiques dans les épilepsies débutant après 60 ans.
Sem. Hôp. Paris 46, 3133-3137 (1970).
VOGEL, F.: Über die Erblichkeit des normalen Elektroenzephalo-
gramms. Stuttgart: Thieme 1958.
VOGEL, F.: Ergänzende Untersuchungen zur Genetik des menschli-
chen Niederspannungs-EEG. Dtsch. Z. Nervenheilk. 184, 105-
111 (1962).
VOGEL, F., GÖTZE, W.: Familienuntersuchungen zur Genetik des
normalen Elektroencephalogramms. Dtsch. Z. Nervenheilk. 178,
668-700 (1959).
VOGEL, F., GÖTZE, W.: Statistische Betrachtungen über die β-
Wellen im EEG des Menschen. Dtsch. Z. Nervenheilk. 184, 112-
136 (1962).
VOGEL, F., GÖTZE, W., KUBICKI, S.: Der Wert von Familienuntersuchungen für die Beurteilung des Niederspannungs-EEG nach
geschlossenem Schädelhirntrauma. Dtsch. Z. Nervenheilk. 182,
337-354 (1961b).
VOGEL, F., WENDT, G.G., OEPEN, H.: Das EEG und das Problem
einer Frühdiagnose der Chorea Huntington. Dtsch. Z. Nervenheilk. 182, 355-361 (1961a).

WADA, T., LENNOX, W.G.: So-called "temporal" epilepsy. The clinical and interseizure EEG-findings. Folia psychiat. neurol. jap. 8, 294-301 (1954).

WHITE, P.T., BAILEY, A.A., BICKFORD, R.G.: Epileptic disorders in the aged. Neurology (Minneap.) 3, 674-678 (1953).

WOODCOCK, S., COSGROVE, J.B.R.: Epilepsy after the age of 50. A five-year follow-up study. Neurology (Minneap.) 14, 34-40 (1964).

YOSHII, N.: Electroencephalographic observation of apparently normal aged subjects. Tokushima J. exp. Med. 103, 203-215 (1971).

YOSHII, N., MATSUMOTO, K., OSHIDA, K.: Clinico-electroencephalographic study of 3200 head injury cases; a comparative work between aged, adults and children. Keiô J. Med. 19, 31-46 (1970).

ZAPPERT, J.: Die Epilepsie im Kindesalter. Ergebn. inn. Med. Kinderheilk. 43, 149-159 (1932).

Subject Index

Schriftenreihe Neurologie – Neurology Series

Herausgeber: H.J. BAUER, H. GÄNSHIRT, P. VOGEL

Springer-Verlag Berlin Heidelberg New York

Clinical Pharmacology of Anti-Epileptic Drugs

International Symposium, Workshop on the Determination of Anti-Epileptic Drugs in Body Fluid II (WODADIBOF II) Held in Bethel, Bielefeld, Germany, 24–25 May 1974. Editors: H. Schneider, D. Janz, C. Gardner-Thorpe, H. Meinardi, A. L. Sherwin

Contents: Pharmacokinetics – Pharmacology of Anti-Epileptic Drugs. – Various Aspects (Varia). – Quality Control and Standardization. – Methodology of Determination. – Dictionary of Anti-Epileptic Drug Synonyms, Chemical Names and Nonproprietary Names. Subject Index.

The proceedings of the Bethel meeting, apart from giving a record and naturally emphasizing the more recently introduced drugs, supplement the currently available reference books on the subject. The volume contributes to present knowledge about anti-epileptic drugs, gives the latest findings and theories on their pharmacokinetics, clinical pharmacology and evaluation as well as advances in analytical methods and presents controversial points of view discussed by experts in the field. This manual is intended as a tool for both the clinician and the scientific worker in pharmacology, epileptology, neurology, pediatrics and neurophysiology as they relate to epileptic disorders. It serves not only to expand and augment knowledge about anti-epileptic drugs but should also improve the treatment of epilepsy patients by basing therapy to a greater extent than hitherto on pharmacokinetic principles.

Springer-Verlag
Berlin
Heidelberg
New York

Printed by Publishers' Graphics LLC